Exercise?

But I Don't Want to!

The Motivated Mover Method **for Women**

By Cathy Dean
Martha Beck Life Coach Cadet
NASM Certified Personal Trainer
ACE Group Fit Instructor

Editing by Meredith Linden
Cover design by Lori Mayo
Printed by CreateSpace

For special sales, contact Cathy Dean at cathymdean@gmail.com.

ISBN: 1492815837
ISBN 13: 9781492815839

Dedicated to Melissa.

Table of Contents

Introduction

In 2011, my two friends died. One in February. One in April. They were my age. Their deaths sent a shockwave through my life. In the months that followed, I cried every day. I quit my job as a personal trainer. I watched a lot of TV. I smoked a lot of cigarettes.

There were days when I couldn't even imagine going to the gym or exercising. But, to my surprise, I exercised every week, which was a lot for being so sad. It wasn't because I wanted to lose weight; I couldn't have cared less about how I looked then. I exercised simply because I was so desperate to *feel* better.

It was the promise of relief. I thought that maybe, if I just moved even for a half hour, I would feel a lightening of the load I was carrying.

I went to the gym a few times on my own, but I felt more empty and alone than ever before. So, I asked my friends to come with me. They got me to the gym when I lacked energy and motivation. Every time I exercised, I felt better. The more I exercised, the easier it was to go back for more. I started going on long walks. Even if a week went by between exercise activities, I still, almost as if on autopilot, found my way back to it.

What kind of motivation lingers even in grief? What kind of energy or sense of self can keep a woman moving even in her darkest hour? What's more, if you had the same set of thoughts and tools to rely on to motivate you in whatever state your life was in, wouldn't you want to know them and use them, too?

When your friend dies, when you lose your job, or when you're really stressed out, what will keep you exercising? Will it be the weight-loss diet with its restrictive meals and vigorous exercise regimen? Or will it be the simple truth that moving your body might offer you some relief from your suffering and maybe even (dare I say it?) pleasure?

Most personal trainers are very good at being structured and restrictive. They thrive in that kind of challenging environment. But I became a personal trainer exactly because I don't thrive with restriction, and most people don't thrive when restricted either. I wanted to show that there was another way to approach fitness. A more intuitive, moderate approach.

You see, motivation to exercise cannot come from discipline alone, which is why I wrote this book. A part is missing from most fitness books out there: it's the part about how to get and keep your motivation to exercise.

I believe in balanced intuitive eating and intuitive exercise. I do not diet. I do not work out to lose weight (though admittedly at times I am still tempted by those quick-fix empty promises). I try to eat the foods that make my body happy. I participate in activities that make me happy like tennis, zumba, yoga, modern dance, walking. Sometimes, when I feel like it, I go to the gym. I eat McDonald's French fries and Oreo cookies. I enjoy wine. I know how it feels to sit on the "sidelines" and wonder how it would feel to be able to run five miles without gasping for air or getting shin splints. Or how crazy it is to fit exercise into your full schedule.

This book's method might not be the route you initially thought you'd take, but the results will be maintainable, and you'll get to enjoy many rewards, including better sleep, improved mood and self-esteem, reduced levels of stress, increased energy, a strengthened heart, and decreased blood pressure, to name a few.

What is the Exercising Magic Formula?

Most fitness books address the technical aspects of performing exercise vigorously (usually for weight loss), but not the details about how to get yourself started, how to have fun, and how to keep yourself going. What good is a fitness program if you never get out of the house to try it? Or can't sustain it?

The magic formula is this: 1) if you participate in an activity you enjoy immensely, you will return to it repeatedly because you get pleasure from it. 2) Even if you love the activity, occasionally, you will have to learn to ignore your excuses, and do it anyway because you know that when you're finished you'll *feel* better.

If you only manage to take away those two ideas, you will be well on your way to gaining and keeping exercise motivation. If you actually apply them to your own life, you're gonna love it!

How It's Gonna Go Down

This book is arranged by tips. The first half are tips to help you ignore your excuses and get you to choose and participate in fun exercise activities. The second half are tips to maintain your exercising once you've started.

If some of the tips don't work for you, don't fret (and don't blame yourself; I give you permission to blame me). Go ahead and move on. Not every tip will fit your needs. So take what makes sense to you and use it.

In spite of the serious beginning to this book, the rest of these pages are lighthearted and easy reading.

These are the tips I have gathered as I looked for ways to stay motivated to exercise. I have included stories of friends and family who have struggled to fit exercise into their lives, sometimes succeeding, sometimes not. (Some of these stories are composites of different people's experiences. Unless permission was granted, names have been changed.) I hope their humble stories and this book help you find your way to intuitive exercise, too.

So what now, you ask?

Simple. All you have to do is turn the page to begin.

PART 1
Getting Away from the Couch

TIP #1

Embrace Your Inner Athlete...

Even If She Likes the Couch More Than Cardio

In this chapter, we're going to find our inner athlete.

Did you laugh out loud there?

Some of you might feel you've never had an inner athlete. If you haven't, that's no problem; now's the time to find her.

So why are we searching for an inner athlete? Simple. We want to tap into our inner athlete so we can find the movement activities we LOVE doing.

When I say inner athlete, I don't mean a professional athlete. A lot of us will never be that serious about movement. Instead, your inner athlete is the part of you that finds joy in exercising and the feeling of activity in your body. Your inner athlete appears when you're playing a game or a sport, or even walking with friends. It appears when you're having fun. In that moment, you might not notice you're moving. When you do notice, you might smile because it feels good. Nothing increases exercise motivation like enjoying the exercise you're doing!

I recently heard this at the gym: "The best part of jogging is stopping." Sound familiar? For many of us, our inner athletes don't come alive with jogging, but we push through because it's convenient. We think we're supposed to jog.

Convenience is only one characteristic of lifetime activities. If the best thing we like about an activity is the end, we can do ourselves a big favor by finding a new activity that enlivens our inner athlete. We need an activity where we say, "The best part about this activity is that I get to do it every day."

Good gravy! Seems like a tall order, doesn't it? Does it make you want to sit on the couch, watch TV and give up?

Go ahead then.

But wait, before you close this book up. Consider this. You started reading this book because doing the same old thing wasn't working for you. Something was missing. Right? Was it your energy? Your excitement for life? That feeling of health in your body?

You've come this far. Why not give it a go? You might find a movement activity that awakens the inner athlete of yours and transforms your life.

The next step is choosing several activities that make us incredibly happy. Let's imagine we're in high school again (oh, the horrors!) or farther back to elementary school.

What kind of movement activities did you enjoy? Take a look at the list and check which ones made you happy.

☐ kickball
☐ four square
☐ hula hoops
☐ monkey bars
☐ gymnastics
☐ soccer
☐ baseball
☐ basketball
☐ dance
☐ football
☐ cheerleading
☐ biking
☐ swimming

☐ track
☐ hockey
☐ rugby
☐ martial arts
☐ walking/hiking
☐ rock climbing
☐ trampolining
☐ skiing or snow-boarding
☐ lifting weights/gym
☐ skating
☐ horseback riding
☐ diving

How'd you feel when you read the list? Did any of these activities spark fond memories for you?

They could have just as easily sparked bad memories for you. This is your chance to change them. Did someone make fun of you because you weren't the best softball player? Fie on them! But that doesn't mean you can't have fun playing softball now. At this point, you're not aiming for perfection or professionalism, you're aiming for fun!

This list can guide you on the path to reawakening your inner athlete and finding your favorite movement activities (and the long-term motivation to exercise).

For example, in high school, I was a cheerleader (you might start to get that vibe from all the exclamation points in this book.). I'm a motivator at heart, and absolutely love dancing. Not only do I like dance, but I like any type of activity where the placement of my body and balance are very important, like Tai Chi and yoga. Those types of activities are endlessly fun for me. They distract me from my burning muscles, which brings me to another point. We can choose exercises for convenience, but I assure you that involving your brain is better. For example, I have discovered I love tennis. Even though I'm really bad at it, I like that I'm trying to be strategic about where to place the ball. Of course, it doesn't mean the ball goes where I intend it to. But it's fun to try.

Let's look at the gym. The elliptical machine or treadmill is definitely convenient, especially during winter time or when it's too hot outside. And there are ways to make the gym fun—go with friends, try one of the preset cardio programs, attend a class, get a personal trainer, or set a personal goal for yourself to go a certain distance or exercise at a certain resistance. But most of us at the gym are exercising our bodies, but not our brains. We're often bored and focused on our discomfort.

I recommend finding an entertaining exercise activity to supplement your time at the gym (if you go to the gym currently). I don't want you to get the impression that I hate the gym. I just know that it's easy to get bored or burnt out at the gym. Spicing it up will help you get moving in all of your activities!

And on the days when you don't feel like going to the gym, you can rely on your supplemental exercise activity of choice to get you away from the couch.

ACTIVITY CHOICE: Why not take a moment right now to make a list of your favorite movement activities. Include ones you did as a kid, the movement activities you've enjoyed in the past few years, and anything you've always wanted to try but thought it was crazy.

Did you write something? Don't worry if you didn't participate in many activities as a kid. This is your time to try now. This is your moment to discover the hidden athlete within.

No groaning! If you don't think you have a hidden athlete within you, if you never liked sports growing up, don't worry. You probably haven't found your special movement activity yet.

What if someone gave you a gift of magic shoes that gave you energy you've never felt before, along with complete body confidence and coordination. Which movement activity would you like to try?

If one comes to mind, put it on the list.

Dr. Richard Wiseman, author of the *The Luck Factor* (2003 Hyperion) emphasizes that people increase their "luck" by increasing the number of times they are exposed to lucky opportunities. Like lucky people, motivated movers increase their chance of finding their favorite activities by increasing their exposure to all different types of activities.

How many have you tried?

So how does the list look? Have you written down everything? Make sure you write down everything you can think of. There's a list in Appendix I to give you more possibilities.

Get creative. Get zany.

Now, without thinking too much about it, circle the one on your list that excites you the most. This is the one you're going to try this very week or even this very day if possible. If you got excited and a little afraid, good. It means we're on the right track.

If you groaned and said, "Oh great," (but said it really sarcastically) then work on your list until you find one that makes you excited.

If you are embarrassed or too timid, consider doing your activity at home. Normally I don't encourage home exercise because for most people, it's harder to maintain. Home is for relaxing. But if there's no way you'll go outside of your home to exercise, home it is!

If you are a large person, want to swim, but hate the swimsuit, there are groups in many areas that offer movement classes for large men and women—dance, swimming, aerobics, yoga, you name it. The National Institutes of Health has a booklet you can access called Active at Every Size that can help you get started. Check out Appendix II for the Web site url and other resources.

Is it just me or are you hesitating a little on making your list? If you haven't done it, please get out a piece of paper and find a movement activity to try!

My friend Lua is my inspiration for this chapter. Whenever she goes running now, she draws from her high school track experience. She taps into her prior knowledge of proper technique. She reminds herself that after a month and a half of hard training, she won't be as sore as she was in the beginning. She also tries to remind herself of her strong inner athlete when doing sprint exercises. Tapping into her inner athlete REALLY motivates her. And the same can happen for you.

Trying Something New—Adventure is Right at Your Back Door!

Sometimes it's scary trying something new. But you can reap plenty of rewards, if only you give it a try.

My friend Janet is a good example of someone who has tried a lot of new activities. She joined an aerobics trampoline class, looked into virtual sky diving, tried rock climbing, kickball, biking, walking, running, and the gym. Being open to new activities gave her the variety she needed to not get bored.

ACTIVITY CHOICE: Trying new things is a great way to keep your excitement about moving at a high level. Have you ever tried trampolining, or lap swimming with fins, or speed walking or skipping? Now is a great time to try it. Add to your list any activities you've always wanted to try but have been too scared to do.

How will you know when you've gotten a good activity? Let me give you an example. I recently was watching the TV show NCIS with my dad and my younger brother. The channel was posting ads at the bottom third of the screen during the show. Dancing people. During the episode, I was so focused on the show, I did not even notice them. I do remember feeling annoyed, like I couldn't really "get" the whole picture at one point, but I never actually saw the ads. My brother noticed every time. Dad noticed half the time. I was fully engaged. That's how you want to be with exercise. Fully distracted from the pain and fully engaged in the activity.

So, find something that makes you forget everything else. Find something that makes you say, "Oh, wow, was I just exercising?"

That's like my friend Tiffany. She really doesn't like the elliptical machine because she knows she's exercising the whole time. Basically, she hates it. But, that's why she likes the Wii and kickboxing. It helps her forget she's exercising. She still does the elliptical for the aerobic challenge, but she prefers more distraction.

What Can Fun Movement Activities Do For Us? They Make Us Forget That Pain in Our Side, Silly!

I really wanted to emphasize the importance of finding a fun movement activity. So here are some reasons why.

It turns out joy can have a big effect on pain. Researchers have done many studies on the effect of laughter in relieving pain. In the journal *Activities, Adaptation & Aging* (Volume 8, Issue 3-4, 1986), researchers Elizabeth R. Adams and Francis A. McGuire studied elderly residents in a long-term care facility. One group of residents watched funny movies, while another group did not. The group that watched funny movies week after week exhibited a decrease in perceived pain.

Joy, and specifically laughter, can also relieve your stress. That's because laughter appears to reduce the levels of hormones creating a stress response in your body, according to a study published in *The American Journal of Medical Sciences* (Dec 1989, Vol 298, Issue 6). The Association for Applied and Therapeutic Humor says laughter increases pain tolerance and counteracts depression and anxiety.

See, there's an inner strength to fun, joyful movement. That's why it's so important for us to find something that is fun for us. It reduces our pain and increases our energy and vigor, which makes doing that movement even easier!

What Else Can Fun Movement Activities Do For Us? They Make Us Want to Do Them Again!

Remember how I said fun was sustainable? Think about it for your own life. What things do you do consistently? How about eating?

We all eat, right? Think about your favorite restaurant. Why do you go? You go again and again because you get a lot of joy from the experience.

Now think about something you thought you should start but didn't. Exercise? Washing the dishes? Or going back to school? For me, it's learning how to read music. As a guitar player, I feel I should know how, but the last time I forced myself to learn, I put the guitar down and didn't pick it up for two years. As soon as I removed the "have to" element of guitar playing, I was playing again. Possibly all you need to do is remove the "have to" thoughts you have about exercise. If you change your exercise approach to fun, you might just become a repeat exerciser.

Many experts—physicians, nurses, sports psychologists and personal trainers—recommend making exercising fun so you'll want to keep doing it.

New exercisers often choose to begin exercising for their health. They internalize the benefits of what exercise will do for them. It's a great way to get yourself started, but I found that for the long-term, balancing exercise-for-health with exercise-for-fun will keep you motivated.

Don't underestimate the emotional aspect of exercising. One study published in the *British Journal of Health Psychology* (Volume 15, Issue 1, pages 1–39, February 2010) divided a bunch of teenagers into two groups. One group received daily text messages about the emotional benefits of exercising (exercising makes you happy). A second group received messages about the physical benefits of exercising (exercising makes your heart stronger). All increased their activity by about 30 minutes per week, but those who received messages about the emotional benefits boosted their exercise activity level by 2 hours per week. Having an emotional motivator—I'll feel happier after I exercise—can get you moving if you let it.

What Else Can Fun Movement Activities Do For Us? They Make Us Healthier.

When we get going with our daily joyful exercising, we can expect some changes to occur. However, we sometimes have trouble recognizing those changes because they happen at the pace of a three-toed sloth.

Look for increased energy levels, improved mood and sense of well-being, along with more strength and flexibility. The stuff you can't feel or see includes reduced risk of the following: Type 2 Diabetes, high blood pressure and cholesterol, heart disease, osteoporosis, arthritis and some cancers (*ACE's Essentials of Exercise Science for Fitness Professionals*, 2012).

Not bad for something you have fun doing!

The Art of Choosing the Right Movement Activity

Did you know that the National Institutes of Health recommends at least 150 minutes of moderate intensity activity or 75 minutes of vigorous activity per week? It's true. And trying to reach those recommendations can be a fun goal. But sometimes people aren't motivated by numbers alone.

They're motivated by fun! And that's often what we're missing when we exercise. We're exercising our bodies, and we forget our brains would like some exercising, too! After a day of sitting in front of a computer, which has made our brains mushy and incapable of focusing, our brains need something fun and stimulating.

Many of us believe certain exercises, like running, are more valid, efficient exercise choices, as if the harder an exercise is, the more valuable it becomes. But here's the truth. *When it comes to being a motivated mover, all movement activities are equally valid.* I don't care what you hear about calories and energy expenditure. An activity you love so much you'll do it for the rest of your life is as valid as setting a goal to run a marathon. Do what you love and ignore anyone telling you different.

I forget sometimes. I had to convince myself as I got wrapped up in researching for this book and in writing these chapters that these fun activities for me are valid activities. I don't know which Puritan in my family instilled the hard-work-before-play ethic, but I have a feeling many of you have the same kind of thoughts roaming in your head.

Let me give you an example of this "fun is not valid" philosophy. My friend Jenn chose to study biology. She worked hard at biology because she knew accomplishing something so difficult would help her feel respected in a career. Halfway through her program though, she realized her heart wasn't in it. She knew she should finish the program, but she couldn't muster up the energy. Finally, she switched to graphic design and marketing—what she loved doing—and gained a sustainable excitement and energy that biology just couldn't provide.

Fun is valid. It is more important than all the data I can throw at you. Fun keeps you going, and it helps you return to movement when you've been sick or when life gets in the way.

"How Lovely!" The Mentor Effect

Challenging exercise can be fun, too. But it helps if you have guidance. In February 2009, I decided I would attend Bikram Yoga in Santiago, Chile—I was living abroad for a year there. Bikram, for those of you who don't know, is hot yoga, performed in a room at 105 degrees F and 40% humidity. Through a series of poses, you sweat like a pig, stretch, and strengthen your muscles and circulatory system. It is somewhere between torture and pleasure. It's the most in-your-face-no-distraction-from-the-sweating-and-stretching exercise out there. I affectionately call it military yoga.

After my first class, I described the experience to a Chilean yoga instructor friend. She responded, "Ah, que rico" which loosely translates to "How lovely!"

I paused for a couple of beats and laughed. I really didn't find Bikram Yoga all that "rico." I felt really good after the class. But the experience in class was really difficult.

Most of all, I was surprised by her response. It got me thinking about the importance of having mentors who can support us in trying new movement activities. Often when we start a new activity, our muscles aren't used to the movement. We feel awkward or ungainly or silly. Then later we feel sore. It's not the most pleasant experience.

Where are the rewards? What keeps us returning? Sometimes, until we get comfortable with a new activity, having someone guide us through the beginning is crucial. A guide or mentor can reveal to us better techniques and better ways of thinking.

Think about it. If I had thought, "que rico" before every Bikram class, during the class and after, I might have become more consistent with yoga in Chile like my friend. But instead, I thought about the heat and the possibility of fainting in class.

I once asked a marathon runner why she liked running so much. She said, "I like it because anyone can improve at it. It doesn't require special talent to run. You just do it." Strangely enough, this simple thought was enough to get me running. I ran all summer, discovered I actually really liked it, and when my roommates came back from vacation, they were incredibly surprised to see I was suddenly a runner.

So if you're having trouble tapping into your inner athlete, you can tap into someone else's inner athlete until you get the hang of your movement activity. Talking to your friends and people you know about your new movement activity will inspire you.

What you'll get from a mentor is someone to show you the ropes and change your perspective. To be a motivated mover, you've got to think like a motivated mover and to do that, you need support from someone who already IS a motivated mover.

You might also get a little envious or intimidated with a mentor as well. It happened to me all the time when I was a personal trainer. There is always someone more fit, stronger, thinner, better, you name it! Allow those thoughts to be there; they're only natural. Your mentor had to be a beginner at one time, too. Approach working with your mentor as a learning experience. Ignore those intimidation feelings and jump right in!

ACTIVITY CHOICE: Please finalize your list of movement activities you'd like to try. Pull from the lists you have created in this chapter. Narrow it down to one you'll try this week (because you're so excited about the prospect of trying it, not because I'm forcing you).

Talk to friends, look on the Internet, go to the library, do whatever it takes to get yourself to do the activity, even if you only try it for 10 seconds and discover it's not for you. Who knows, you might discover it's the thing you've been missing from your life.

If you discover it isn't for you, take the next movement activity on your list that looks interesting to you and try that. It's time to awaken your inner athlete and harness that exercise motivation!

Motivated Mover Activities to Try Today or Right Now to Embrace Your Inner Athlete

---

ACTIVITY CHOICE: Go back through the chapter and do the activities if you haven't done them yet.

ACTIVITY CHOICE: Pick a mentor who does the movement activity you want to try (or who is adventurous and willing to try it with you) and call them right now.

ACTIVITY CHOICE: Go to your activity of choice.

TIP #2

Get to Know
(and Become) Your
Exercise Self

A key element to becoming a motivated mover is understanding how you function with and react to exercise. The people most successful at consistent exercise know how they behave with the thought of exercise and use that information to keep going.

It's kind of like setting your clocks ahead if you know you always run a bit late.

That's what this chapter is all about. Figuring out how you react faced with the prospect of exercise.

Take the following quiz to find out what your exercise style most closely resembles. Circle the questions to which you answer "yes" or take note of your "yes's" on a separate piece of paper. Since no one but you is going to see this, why not admit what exercise is really like for you?

Quiz 1: Exercise Style

1. Do you dread exercise time but exercise anyway because you know it's good for you?

2. Do you put off exercising for as long as possible, sometimes for months or years?

3. Do you find it's difficult to get started, but once you start, you like to move?

4. Are you determined to do whatever movement activity it takes to accomplish your goal, even if you don't like the movement activity you're doing?

5. Do you find it's easy to motivate yourself to exercise in the short term, say a month, but you can't seem to stay consistent throughout a year's time?

6. Have you ever injured yourself from overdoing it?

7. Would you rather play the Wii than go to the gym?

8. Do you love sports?

9. Do you love the feeling of winning?

10. Have you given up on movement altogether?

11. Do you feel so embarrassed exercising in front of other people that you don't even want to think about exercising?

12. Are you bored but mostly consistent with your movement routine?

13. Are you only exercising to prevent an injury or because the doctor told you to?

Don't be shy. Circle away. Write directly on the book.

On the following pages, you'll find five "exercise styles" that correspond to the questions you answered. Each section describes the style and possible solutions to finding and maintaining enthusiasm for exercise.

Take a look and pick out which style best describes you. You might find you connect with more than one style, which is fine. Read the solutions, come up with your own, too, and apply your favorites to your life.

Slow-Starter: (yes to 1, 2, 3)

DESCRIPTION: Slow starters like you don't mind exercise...all that much. You understand the benefits of exercise. You want to exercise (you think), but you just can't seem to get started.

EXERCISE BARRIERS: Beginning exercise feels like a gargantuan effort. You are also very susceptible to any break in your routine which will often derail your exercise completely. Any break becomes then another terrible climb to start again.

NEEDS: Use this knowledge about yourself to overcome "starting-is-impossible" thinking. If you're interested in a gym environment, a personal trainer can show you the ropes. What you need more than anything are activities you enjoy doing for pleasure, instead of viewing exercise as a punishment. Find something that has always been fun for you and focus on doing that fun activity more than anything else.

Slow-starters like you can also use a perspective change from thinking exercise is merely a six-week program. We'll talk more about changing from program to lifestyle thinking in future chapters (I know you're excited!).

Ask a friend to go through the following book activities with you if it's hard to do on your own. Acknowledge you need help with getting started, get that help in place and go for it!

Achiever (Yes to 1, 3, 4, 5, 6, 9)

DESCRIPTION: Achievers like you are driven to exercise, to be the best at it, and to do it exactly as recommended by experts. You are very goal-oriented and up for any challenge. You're likely to perform difficult workouts and activities.

EXERCISE BARRIERS: Your ambition can expose you to injury or exhaustion because you may sacrifice the body to accomplish the goal. Your approach can often lead to a dislike of exercise since achievers can begin to view exercise as one more chore on the gigantic to-do list. You may also feel despondent and lost once your goal is accomplished.

NEEDS: A supplement of fun-only movement activities without goals added to your goal-driven exercises can help you find more motivation. If you can't let go of goals (I know! What a crazy idea!), follow the goal approach in Tip #5 to create many sequential goals rather than one goal. Listen to your body to prevent injury.

Maintainer (yes to 1, 3, 4, 12, 13)

DESCRIPTION: Maintainers like you go to the gym to keep at a current health level and to avoid injuries. You have no interest in pushing your body to new fitness levels...or you do, but your interest isn't enough of a motivator to push you to action. Maintainers are consistent over the long term, but allow themselves a lot of days off—for washing their hair, for lazy days, for every bad-day or good-day excuse they can think of.

EXERCISE BARRIER: Boredom with the same old routine after years can lead to avoiding exercising like a cat avoids getting a bath—with a lot of claws and surprising determination.

NEEDS: You could use an exercise invigoration. You like habits a lot so there's no need for a lot of change, but every six months, change movement activities so you're not falling asleep while exercising. If you're a gym-goer, change up your workout routine or hire a personal trainer to show you some new moves.

Gamer (yes to 3, 5, 6, 7, 8, 9)

DESCRIPTION: Gamers like you are goal- and sports-oriented. You like games with a clear objective and a way to win. You do well in team activities and when there's competition. You respond well to training for special events. You like having lots of fun (I mean, who doesn't!).

EXERCISE BARRIERS: You move for fun but you have trouble staying consistent. When the sports season is over, your exercise habits are over, too. You have trouble staying consistent without a game-element to your exercising. If you haven't exercised in years, you've forgotten your love of sports and games and might also identify with the slow-starter style.

NEEDS: You need to have other sports set up to replace the one ending. This will encourage consistent exercise year-round. Or when you're not playing sports, make exercising a game. Invest in an interactive video game console or bring a friend to the gym to compete with for the most reps, heaviest weight lifted or most time on the elliptical machine.

Avoider (yes to 2, 6, 10, 11)

DESCRIPTION: Avoiders like you hate moving and have had serious issues with movement in the past. You might feel totally uncomfortable in your body. You don't like sweating (ew gross!), and you feel embarrassed by how much you sweat. You don't like the feeling of breathing heavily either. You ignore your body signals or don't even realize what your body is telling you (don't worry, you're just out of practice). You would do anything to avoid moving. If you use the excuse "I need to get fit before I exercise" then this style might resonate with you.

EXERCISE BARRIERS: Your biggest barrier to exercise is fear. Your past experiences have led you to believe that exercise is a painful, embarrassing, or nausea-inducing experience (it can be, but it doesn't have to be).

NEEDS: First, you might need to boost your body image. Start by going through the baby steps in the bonus tip in the back of the book. Look online for other body image exercises. Also, think about exercise as a vehicle to help you share in more activities with friends, family and your children. Being active with others can be a powerful motivator. Finding the right activity that fits you is important. Find an activity that makes you feel good and aware of your body, and is in a safe environment, with good people, and at the right time. Being accountable to an exercise buddy can also help you tremendously.

All these styles have great qualities about them and distinct barriers that prevent these types from becoming motivated movers. Which one(s) do you identify with?

ACTIVITY CHOICE: Now go back to the descriptions and the needs of your style(s). Think about where you've gotten stuck in the past and how you can preempt that behavior this time. Knowledge is power. When your mind resists (out of habit), you can proactively shift gears and get motivated to exercise anyway.

Write your ideas in a notebook or somewhere where you can review them frequently.

Quiz 2: Energy Levels—
When is Your Best Time to Exercise?

Now that you have an idea about your exercise style, we come to circadian rhythms. It's another important part of knowing your exercise self.

Take my brother's story for example. My younger brother was trying to start a consistent weight-lifting and running program. But he was soon frustrated. No matter how hard he tried, he couldn't convince himself to get up before work to exercise.

I shared with him my own inability to get up to exercise in the mornings—it turns out that I'd rather sleep than exercise. Every few years (recently even!) I try to exercise in the mornings. Exercise makes me happy, so I logically assume I should exercise as soon as possible in the day to maximize my happiness. This logic is lost on me in the morning. I snooze and sleep right through exercise time.

My brother decided, since he liked to stay up late at night, a workout at 10pm or 11pm might flow better with his natural energy cycle. And sure enough, it worked!

What had been a struggle before turned into consistent exercise. Two and a half years later, my brother was still exercising two to three days a week, a consistency he struggled to achieve with his early morning workout attempts. More recently, he has been playing basketball after work, an activity he has enjoyed since high school.

Now it's your turn. So let's discover when your best time of the day for exercise is. Answer morning, afternoon, or evening to each question.

1. What time of day do you most need caffeine or feel tired?
2. What time of day do you feel grumpiest?
3. What time of day do you feel happiest?
4. If you were to do something creative, when would you do it?
5. Think of a time when you felt you were most consistent with exercise. What time of day did you exercise?
6. What time of day would be the least interrupted by life (family, friends, chores, work)?

The answers to 1 and 2 indicate when you're at your lowest energy point. This can be a good time for you to re-energize and clear your head, especially if it's relatively easy for you to convince yourself to exercise. Gamers and overachievers are good candidates for exercising at their lowest energy points if they so choose because they already have a higher motivation to exercise.

Answers to 3 and 4 indicate when your highest energy levels happen. If you have trouble with motivating yourself to get started, exercising at your highest energy levels can help you establish consistency, a consistency you struggle to achieve when exercising at your lowest energy levels. Maintainers, Avoiders and Slow-Starters can benefit from exercising at their highest energy levels.

The answer to 5 can be very revealing. Consistent exercisers work with who they are to make exercise a larger part of their lives. Look at situations in the past that have worked the best for you. If you were most consistent in the morning, for example, consider starting a morning movement activity. Go with what works for you.

And the last answer. Life is busy, and chores, family, jobs and more can interrupt your plans to exercise if you let them or if you're susceptible to allowing interruptions to derail your exercise plans. If you're a slow-starter, avoider, or maintainer, schedule exercise to happen in those blocks of time least likely to get interrupted by life. This might mean that even though you're not a morning person, your best chance to fit in exercise might be before work (because no one else is crazy enough to get up that early).

Though we may not be able to line up our lives exactly with our energy levels, we can align them better. For example, if you decided afternoon is when you're most willing to exercise but you work until 6pm, ask your boss to adjust your schedule. If that doesn't work, exercise during lunch. There are options. If you do have an activity that doesn't align with the timing of your energy levels, make sure it is the most fun activity on the planet! Sometimes you can overcome non-exercise energy times with the promise of a fun time.

Incidentally, you can apply this idea to other parts of your life. If you have any control on when you do the more creative or demanding aspects of your job, consider doing them when you have the most energy to get the most out of your natural energy cycles.

ACTIVITY CHOICE: Now that you know this information, what time of day would work best to exercise? Write down in your notebook when you plan to exercise and why.

Look back at your answer to number 5 of the energy levels quiz. Besides energy levels, what was it that encouraged your most consistent movement? Did you exercise with friends? Was it a class that kept you most consistent? If it was part of a short-term program, what part can you adapt for your purposes here? Was it a fun type of activity that kept you going? Was it a feeling of energy? Was it the rewards? Or the progress you felt?

Note your answers in your notebook and keep them as we continue getting to know our mover selves.

Quiz 3: To Be with People or to Go it Alone

I know you know you, but if you're reading this book, you might not know the "exercise you." One key element to exercising is knowing whether you like exercising with other people or whether it makes you cringe.

I'm a little shy but find I enjoy exercising with people a lot more than on my own, especially weight lifting. I cannot, for the life of me, get myself to enjoy weight lifting on my own—and I was a personal trainer for goodness sakes! So for me, even though I'm shy, I prefer people. That's why classes or working out with friends are the best fits for me.

Find out for yourself (if you don't already know) which exercise preference works best for you.

1. Do you enjoy being with people more than being by yourself?
2. Do you get really excited and high energy when you're with people?
3. Are you more interested in doing team sports like soccer than solo sports like running or ice skating?
4. Do you rely heavily on others to keep you motivated?
5. Do you feel anxious and shy around people?
6. Do you feel uncomfortable exercising in front of other people?
7. Do you prefer to not have attention from others?
8. Does your own ambition drive you?

A yes to questions 1 through 4 shows an inclination to be with people. A yes to questions 5-8 show an inclination to go it alone.

ACTIVITY CHOICE: Write down in your notebook whether you'll search for activities with people or go it alone.

Exercising with friends, teammates or classmates can be really fun. It contributes to your overall energy during the activity and consistency in returning. But it all depends on you. If the idea of sweating in front of anyone gives you chills (the horror kind, not the excitement kind), then group classes and team sports might not be for you. That's a-okay.

Solutions for the loners: Buy new exercise videos. Try walking, running or biking on your own. Find a personal trainer who offers sessions at their private gym, at your home or outside in the park. Or ask your friends for teachers who might offer private lessons in your movement activity of choice.

My friend Kelley took private Tai Chi lessons for 10 years. Kelley hates crowds. He prefers intimate gatherings to parties. He doesn't mind classes, but the combination of his energy level (morning/afternoon), his "no people" preference, his maintainer style due to injuries, and his love for Tai Chi meant the private Tai Chi lessons at noon were perfect for him. He set himself up for movement success, and the only reason he stopped was because his teacher moved away. When that happened, he began teaching Tai Chi to me!

Quiz 4: Structured Goals or Flexible Purpose

My dad mentioned to me once that he couldn't set physical exercise goals that lasted longer than three months. He liked structure but he got bored by it, too. For him, a short-term structured goal is the answer.

Now it's your turn to discover what works best for you. Answer the questions below:

1. Are you a creature of habit?
2. Do you thrive when you have a clear set of rules to follow?
3. Do you enjoy fitness programs because someone else is telling you what and when you should be doing your activity?
4. Do you enjoy going to movement classes because they follow a pattern?
5. Do you get bored easily with the same old routine?
6. Do you feel trapped when you have to follow a lot of techniques or rules?
7. Do you rebel against set programs and plans you have to follow?
8. Do you find it hard to form a long-term exercise habit because you can't seem to do it for more than 4-6 weeks before you start to feel antsy, bored, rebellious or annoyed?

If you answered yes to 1-4, you respond better to structure. Classes, rules, programs all help you stay focused and interested. Try establishing an exercise schedule to form a comfortable habit. You can take a look at Tip #5 to help you set clear goals.

If you answered yes to 5-8, you respond better to a more flexible approach. The time you exercise doesn't need to be the same every day. Choose many sequential short-term activities to keep from getting bored or rebelling from the same old routine.

ACTIVITY CHOICE: Write your preferred exercise approach (structured or flexible) in your notebook. If you have characteristics of both, write them both down and incorporate suggestions from both approaches into your movement activities.

Let's State the Obvious

Do you like or hate the gym?

This is definitely an important question. If you like the gym, great! The gym can be really convenient and a good way to de-stress.

If you hate the gym, it probably isn't the place for you. It just isn't your thing. No big deal.

But have you actually tried it? Have you gone with friends who are gym rats? I would highly recommend getting a guest pass, going with friends and trying it out.

If you already have a habit of going to the gym, don't give that up for this book. Your hatred for the gym can stem from boredom. Get a book on exercises (look at Tip #8 for one such routine), and shake up what you always do. Just add other more exciting activities to do every other day.

Oh, just one thing to consider. It's very possible what you don't like is the TYPE of gym where you exercised. You might have gone to a 24 Hour Fitness but your style might fit Curves more. Or you could prefer a swim and racquet club. Who knows? The YMCA could be your place.

Before you completely write off the gym, ask your friends if they have a favorite gym and why. It can't hurt to check it out, right? We'll talk more about choosing a gym in Tip #8.

So now that we've taken the quizzes, what do we do with them?

What Can Knowing Ourselves Do For Us?

Knowing ourselves can help us get to our exercise activity. You can find the movement activity that will fit you best if you know what you like and don't like.

Take my friend Dana, for instance. She was looking for something to remove some of her stress. She had a busy life with two children, a husband, and a thriving massage therapy practice. She had tried exercising in her home but the distractions of home prevented her from making it a habit. Plus those exercises didn't speak to her soul. As she figured out more and more about what she wanted and needed in a movement activity, she found her way to yoga. The activity fits with her values, her heart and her soul.

Lua, on the other hand, makes up drum rhythms all the time in her head. She loves pushing herself and participating in challenging workouts. For her, African dance with live drumming matched very well with her heart, mind and spirit. African dance satisfies her need for something physically challenging, soulful and rhythmic.

How Do You Know When You've Found the Right Movement Activity?

I believe everyone has the movement activity that speaks to them, that goes right to their souls. How do you know when you've found yours? Well, long-lasting excitement or pride at a job well done usually shows up. Sometimes you can't stop smiling through it. And when you're finished you might be tired, but you are also excited. You can't help talking about it with your friends and boring them to tears.

Motivated Mover Activities to Try
Today or Right Now to Know (and Become)
Our Exercise Selves

ACTIVITY CHOICE: Look back at your answers to these quizzes. Review what you have learned about your exercise self and write down the final summary. What's your exercise style? Your natural energy rhythm? Your people preferences? Your preferred exercise quality (structured/flexible)? Your feelings about the gym? Sum it up.

Now that you know your exercise self, it's time to become it! Keep reading to begin your lifelong love affair with fitness!

TIP #3

Still Having Trouble Getting Started? Recharge Your Qi!

Are you still having trouble getting started? Can't seem to muster up the energy for it? This chapter is just for you! If you are already going to movement activities, then go ahead and skip to the next tip. But if you haven't done the book activities yet, this tip is for you.

Here's a secret for you. Whether you exercise or not is really not a big deal. Truth is, you'll still have a solid, valid life if you decide to never exercise again. But I do have to tell you the one simple truth: **your life will be better with exercise in it.**

You'll feel happier, more vigorous and energetic. You'll feel less achy. You'll have more energy. Eventually, you may even have the confidence to go hiking, take that martial arts, yoga or dance class you've always wanted to try, or opt for the stairs instead of the escalator in the mall.

Of course, it's one thing to talk about the benefits of exercise, and quite another to get enough gumption and energy to go and do it. This chapter is here to help you recharge your Qi (pronounced chee) and acquire more energy so getting yourself going won't be such a challenge.

I'm going to start by giving you permission to not exercise...at least not yet. I got the idea from my acupuncturist who tells her low-energy (and sometimes depressed) clients the same thing. Here's why she offers this advice. When her depressed clients confess to feeling guilty for not exercising, she recommends they wait until they feel their body is ready. They will know when it's time to exercise. Then after three or four weeks of acupuncture treatment, her clients start to feel better inside. Their life force or Qi becomes balanced. They have more energy and feel happier. Before they know it, voila, they've cleaned the garage and joined a gym.

"Don't do it...at least not yet" offers us a way out from the "shoulds." Don't make exercise a "should" on your list of chores. When your exercise is a "should," you make it as appealing as wrestling crocodiles...in a bikini!

There will always be days when exercise is going to be the last thing you want to do (maybe that's even today.). **To be able to remind yourself that you don't HAVE to exercise is the first step.** This leaves about an inch of room for exercising to become a want. And every inch helps. After all, it only takes the tiniest crack in a rock for a seed to grow into a plant. **The second and MOST IMPORTANT step is to remind yourself that, somewhere in there, you *want* to exercise.** When you get to a point where you *want* to exercise because you'll *feel* so great afterward in body and mind, getting yourself out the door is much easier.

How Do We Get to the Point Where We'll WANT to Exercise?

Think about a time when you were really, really happy—your happiest moment. Didn't you have tons of energy? Didn't it feel like you could run five marathons or at least down the block and back without breaking a sweat?

It's true. Being happy is a great motivator to go work out. But probably, if you're not exercising, you might not be as happy (or as energetic as you could be). It's a virtuous cycle once you step into it, but it's tough to start. Think about it: Exercise supplies you with endorphins which make you happy...Happiness gives you more energy...More energy gives you motivation to exercise... Exercise makes you happy...and so on!

But how can you jump into that cycle if you're feeling lazy, low-energy or even a little depressed? How do we recharge our Qi or energy without the acupuncture needles? (And by the way, I highly recommend trying acupuncture if you are feeling depressed or low-energy. It works for me!)

One option is to force ourselves to exercise anyway, in spite of having no energy. However, I would bet your success with this approach has been low since you're reading this book. Also, this forcing approach can be the way you develop guilty feelings on top of depressed feelings.

If we can't use needles to boost our energy—and haven't been able to *force* ourselves to exercise—we can at least try an easier technique to boost our happiness and our energy.

In an earlier draft of this book, I had offered meditation as a way to recharge your Qi and regain some of the energy you lack. I still think meditation is a great idea. It certainly helps me clear my head when I'm stressed or depressed. But it's difficult for a lot of people to sit still and pay attention to their breathing.

That's why I'm offering a modified approach. Instead you'll be performing a walking meditation. Meditation doesn't have to be sitting down. It can be anything where you remain focused on the present moment.

However, if you're feeling particularly low-energy, and the walk sounds excruciating, stick with a sitting meditation instead. See Appendix III for meditation instructions. Or you can choose to color (and try collaging or another type of art project). Coloring is easier for some than meditation but offers some of the same benefits: You relax through focusing on the task at hand. Your sense of awareness shifts. You may begin to notice your internal dialogue, and noticing can help you develop that sense of compassion for yourself and others. Pretty soon you'll have recharged your Qi enough to think about other movement activities you'd like to do!

ACTIVITY CHOICE: For those interested in the meditation walk, let's keep it simple. Put on comfortable clothes and shoes, and step out your front door, and start walking. Go your own pace:

slow, vigorous, whatever. As you walk, pay attention to your breath and to what you see, hear and feel. Be in the moment. When your thoughts wander, gently and without judgment bring your attention back to the moment you're in. Walk for at least 10-30 minutes... the amount that feels good to you. Go ahead and do it now if time and weather permit.

When I go on a meditation walk, I like walking for 45 minutes to an hour. It takes that long for my head to clear and to feel that sense of uplift and bounce in my step. Go for the length of time that feels good to you!

If you can't today, schedule it into your day tomorrow. In fact, try to schedule a walk every day for a week. If weather doesn't permit walking outside, head to the gym and walk on the treadmill instead. The goal of this practice is NOT about exercise as much as it is about you learning to pay attention to how your body feels and the thoughts that run through your head—to, in effect, "recharge your Qi."

Notice how you feel when you're finished. Your body might feel warmer, your thoughts might seem clearer, or you might feel more relaxed. You could even feel happier.

Sometimes we don't even notice when our mood improves or when we have slightly more energy than before. I want you to take note of it by keeping an exercise/energy journal for your week of walking. This is for the beginners who have difficulty recognizing how beneficial exercise is to improving your energy and happiness levels.

Exercise Journal

Make a copy of this page. Use it every time you exercise to help you become aware of how your body and mind feel after you've finished.

Date:

What I did and for what amount of time:

How I felt, thought, and acted before I exercised. Why did I exercise? Did I want to exercise?:

My pre-exercise happiness on a scale from 1-10 (10 being most happy):

My pre-exercise energy on a scale from 1-10 (10 being most energetic):

How I felt, thought, and acted after I exercised:

My post-exercise happiness on a scale from 1-10 (10 being most happy):

My post-exercise energy on a scale from 1-10 (10 being most energetic):

What I ate before my workout and how that food helped or hindered my workout:

How I can improve:

You might find that your body feels the same kind of sluggishness before each walk. Are you overly anxious? Are you feeling heavy or sad? Your body has signals for hunger and fullness. I believe there are also "exercise-me" signals. The exercise-me signals vary widely in intensity and range. Some of these signals include feeling sluggish, irritable, grumpy, cloudy in the head, tired, anxious, angry, restless, fidgety, sad or achy. See if you can recognize your own body's pattern and need for exercise. After your walk, take note of how you feel. If you feel the same pre- and post-walk, try to walk for longer the next day.

After a week of walking, you might start to notice an increase in your energy and happiness level, though that increase might be slight. Either continue to walk, or consider rereading the first two chapters and choosing a movement activity besides walking to try. If walking is starting to feel good, and that's all you can muster for now, keep it up. The more you walk, the better you'll feel.

It's like your car when it's covered in dust. Eventually some wise guy gives you the signal by writing "wash me" on the back window. Heed the message by washing your car, and your car looks brand new. You might even think, "Wow, this is my car? I'd like to wash it more often!"

Same goes for your body. Heed the message by moving, and your body rewards you by giving you a feeling of being more "clean and clear." It even rewards you over time in how you move by becoming stronger and more efficient. Ignore the message, and your brain and body feel like they're covered in mud.

Why Are We Doing This Again?

If this has already triggered an existential crisis (or you desperately want to skip ahead but can't seem to stop reading), you probably need a bit more information on how something like a walking meditation and being in the present moment might help you find the motivation for further exercise. It seems like a big leap. It turns out the leap is more like a small skip in the park.

For instance, when you practice meditation, even if it's only for ten breaths, you're reaping many rewards. You're taking a break from your fast-paced, busy life. You're dedicating time to something that's good for you and developing feelings of compassion toward yourself. Sometimes, we berate ourselves for not doing what we should do, when really, we're having a hard enough time keeping up with living. Who has time or energy to work out when we come home each day feeling like a truck ran us over?

By giving ourselves space to breathe with meditation, we can find more energy. We can become a motivated mover.

Meditation is powerful. J. Kabat-Zinn published the results of a mindfulness study in the *Pyschosomatic Medicine Journal* (1998 Sep-Oct;60(5):625-32) related to a group of patients with psoriasis. They split the group into two, and both groups received the current Western treatment, while one group meditated in addition to the normal treatment. Guess which group healed faster? That's right, the meditating group. If meditation can help our body heal faster, why couldn't it help us gather up more energy for moving?

Motivated Mover Activities to Try Today or Right Now to Recharge Your Qi

---

ACTIVITY CHOICE: Walk or meditate every day for a week.

ACTIVITY CHOICE: Focus on a simple task such as coloring or collage. If you liked either of these activities, why not consider doing these activities more often?

ACTIVITY CHOICE: Fill out the Exercise Journal for your walking meditation week. Is it helpful to tune your senses to your energy and happiness levels? Continue if you find it helpful. If not, pay attention to the next chapter on overcoming Lazy Brain.

ACTIVITY CHOICE: Go back and do the activities in the first two tips. Choose an activity to try and go with a friend.

Keep going, you're doing great!

TIP #4

Useful Ways to

Overcome Lazy Brain

I'm glad you have read this far. If you haven't done the activities in this book, go back and do them now. This chapter is more useful to you once you've attended at least a few exercise activities.

Have you ever watched someone trying to quit smoking? They're doing well until a stressful situation occurs, and then they crave a cigarette so much they're willing to sell their grandma for a drag. The situation doesn't necessarily have to be all that stressful, but smokers are looking for any plausible excuse to start smoking. They can't help it. When they find their excuse, they succumb to habit and addiction. I know. I've had to quit many times!

The same happens with exercise, especially when our initial motivation is gone, we've had a bad day or haven't slept well. The unmotivated, low-energy exerciser craves junk food and the couch and their favorite TV series just as strongly as a smoker craves the cigarette.

We become afflicted with lazy brain.

In the same way a smoker unaccustomed to their smoke-free habit looks for an excuse to return to "normal," so does the unmotivated exerciser look for excuses to get back on the couch.

By now, you've identified your exercise self. You've chosen and even tried some of the activities on the list you made. You've recharged your Qi with a meditation walk if you needed that extra boost.

If you haven't already, one day soon, you may become afflicted by lazy brain. Lazy brain is every exerciser's most common affliction—it's the frame of mind where the couch looks great and everything else does not. Lazy brain is one big reason so many people can't stay consistent with exercise.

So what can we do when it appears?

We initiate a preemptive strike—just like we started in the previous chapters with understanding our exercise selves. We basically anticipate our own excuses and make sure we have workable solutions to get ourselves moving.

Pay Attention to Your Excuse Thoughts...without Reacting

Remember how I had you meditate or do the meditation walk? I'm hoping you've continued those relaxation techniques because we're going to need your newfound meditating prowess here.

Just as a reminder, when we meditate (walking or sitting), we can observe our thoughts scurrying by like clouds on a windy day.

It is an opportunity to observe our thoughts without reacting to them...which is hard to do, but useful when we can.

This "observing without reacting" idea is important for combating exercise excuses because over time, we can put a little space between us and our thoughts. When the thought, "I don't want to go exercise," comes up, you can observe without reacting. You might wait a second longer before plopping on the couch, chips in hand. Or you might ignore the thought completely!

Look. Everyone has lazy brain. But not everyone has to listen to it.

Let's first start with the past. What have been some of your excuse patterns with previous fitness programs? Do any of these ring a bell:

1. I'm too tired; I just don't have energy.
2. I'm too stressed.
3. I'm too busy.
4. My kid/husband/dog/hamster needs me.
5. I hurt my pinky and so therefore can't do any movement at all.
6. I'm on vacation.
7. I had a hard day and deserve a break.
8. I'm depressed.
9. I'm too sore.
10. I can't afford it.
11. I need to get fit before I exercise.
12. I was sick last week.
13. I was injured last week. I don't want to risk it.

ACTIVITY CHOICE: Write the excuses you most use in your notebook. If your excuse didn't make my list, write your own.

Excuses are nothing more than signals telling you that you need to provide yourself additional motivation and inspiration. Usually it means you have fearful or distasteful thoughts about exercise. A study in the *Research in Higher Education Journal* (Volume 39, Issue 2, pp 199-215) showed that college students prone to excuse making and procrastination didn't like the task they had to do, were afraid of failing the task, or feared disapproval from peers. You too could have similar reasons for your excuses... and once you know them, you can change them. So check out the three questions below in the context of your exercise excuses:

1. Is the activity I'm going to do fun? Do I generally have a great time when I go?

If yes, continue. If no, choose a different activity.

2. Do I fear I will fail the task?

If yes, work on ways to make yourself less afraid of failure. Achievers often answer yes to this question. It helps to remind ourselves to enjoy our exercise and not to aim for perfection. I also remind myself that those people who look really great at an exercise have most likely been practicing for years. And that someday, if I continue to enjoy that activity, I could also look that great!

For example, look at any "new" actor or actress on the scene, someone who seemingly became famous overnight. With few exceptions, their bio and list of bit parts in movies is usually 10 years in the making!

In Malcolm Gladwell's *Outliers: The Story of Success*, he emphasizes that it takes 10,000 hours to master a skill. So unless you've done this movement activity for 10,000 hours, don't worry about looking new at it. You are!

3. Do I fear people will make fun of me?

I know it's difficult to receive criticism from others, especially nosy, bossy strangers who think it's their business to tell you what to do. But the great thing about being an adult is that you don't have to listen to them, take their advice or even pretend to like them. Just try not to get violent, okay? Ignore them and enjoy your movement activity. The people you're meant to meet and be friends with will show up.

ACTIVITY CHOICE: Think about your fears and aversion behind your excuses. What kind of responses will you tell yourself to counteract those emotions? Write them down so you'll be ready when they come up for real.

Listen, you're the one driving this fitness bus so if you get a lot of excuses coming up in your thoughts, it's possible you haven't chosen the right activity. Search through the list in the Appendix I until you find one that gives you a little spark of happiness or hope. That's the one worth trying.

However, if you think finding the perfect movement activity will get rid of your excuses forever, you're wrong. Even with the promise of an awesome activity, there are just some days when you're going to need a little help getting started.

For example, I absolutely love dance, but I still get a lot of excuse thoughts before every dance class. I **always** have a great time, but still, the excuses come! "It's too far away." "I'm too tired." "I don't want to go." "I'll have to move my body!" "I just want to be at home." To overcome my excuse thoughts, I think about my previous times dancing. No matter how I think beforehand, I am energized and happy every time after. I know that if I can just get myself off the couch and out the door, I'll come back two hours later bouncing off the walls with excitement and energy and feeling really, really good! I ask myself, "Do I want to feel really good and happy?" I answer yes. Then I go to dance class (most of the time). And then I feel good and happy.

And so, try these tricks to counteract your own lazy brain. Though every exercise style may benefit from each trick, I have suggested who may benefit the most from each:

1. As soon as you think about doing your movement activity, put on the outfit. Style: avoider, slow-starter, achiever

Putting on clothes for your movement activity is a declaration to others and to yourself. It says simply, "I intend to exercise." It is a commitment. The small act of putting on my exercise clothes has helped me get to the gym. For me, as an achiever, it's easier to go exercise than to have to face the guilt of failing to follow through.

2. Fall in love with feeling sore. Style: avoider, slow-starter, maintainer

You're going to feel sore. It's inevitable. It's normal. The feeling of soreness a day or two after a movement activity is a result of small tears in your muscles, and is the natural part of exercising, especially if you're performing a new exercise or movement.

Take pride in it. It means you've done something good for your body. Your muscles are growing with each movement activity session. You're getting stronger.

However, for some of you, pride is little compensation when placed side-by-side with the ever-present sore butt, legs or arms. If you're taking the stairs slowly because you're sore from exercising, there are some ways to relieve some of your pain:

Self-Myofascial Release (SMR) with Foam Roller (i.e., self-massage)

Self-myofascial release is a method much like self-massage. Several studies have shown that massages reduce levels of delayed onset muscle soreness associated with exercise, and since massages can be expensive, the foam roller is a cheap alternative.

By applying at least 30 seconds of gentle pressure using your body weight and a foam roller, you can find knots in your muscles and massage them out. It is considered a method for stretching because when knots are released, your muscles can return to their optimal lengths. A NASM workshop trainer described it as the difference in length between a shoestring with five knots in it and a shoestring with none.

Warm Up and Cool Down

If you find your muscles cramping during your movement activity, it can be an indication of several things. You could be lacking nutrients like potassium or sodium, which can be solved by drinking a sports drink, especially if you exercise for more than 60-90 minutes.

It can also be an indication that you need to lengthen your warm up. A warm up, the first 5 or 10 minutes of exercise, should be a gentle increase in intensity. An adequate warm up allows your muscles to slowly adjust to the change in speed, produce energy, draw in more oxygen and pump your heart faster. It also acts as a mental preparation—a kind of "get ready" period of exercise, like the breathing in before blowing out a birthday candle.

The cool down as well can be very effective in preventing muscle cramps and tightening. The cool down is the final 5 or 10 minutes and is marked by a gentle decrease in intensity.

Ice or Heat

Both ice and heat can relieve sore muscles. With ice, the sore area is numbed. When the ice is removed, blood rushes to the area and can facilitate faster healing. Applied heat increases muscle temperature, which increases blood flow, allowing for faster healing.

Ice has been more effective for me than heat—find out which one works best for you!

Stretching

It is not clear that stretching prior to exercise relieves soreness, and certain studies found it did not alleviate soreness at all. But gentle stretching feels good in loosening tight muscles. Stretch if it feels good for you and works for you.

Rest

Since probably only certain muscle groups are sore, try resting those muscle groups and targeting other muscle groups. If your arms are sore, walking or running can be a good activity to get your body in motion without overtaxing your arms.

By the way, if the feeling of pain is sharper, occurs during exercise and is accompanied by inflammation or bruising, it is more likely injury than the normal after-exercise soreness. When that happens, rest is VERY important, as is consulting a doctor should the pain not subside.

Those are just some ways to make after-exercise soreness less of an excuse. I have found that, out of all these options, SMR and warming up have worked best for me in reducing soreness.

I also want to mention another possible way to combat the "pain" excuse. We can often feel achy when we don't exercise at all. For example, I find my body starts to get achy when I don't exercise for a while. So, if the choice is exchanging one type of pain for another, and exercising offers additional benefits such as being a mood enhancer, why not choose the mood-enhancing option?

3. Create an exercise "river current." Style: slow-starter, avoider, gamer (on off-season)

Just like a river current can carry a twig far downstream, an exercise habit can carry a motivated mover effortlessly downstream, too. Anyone who's tried to break a habit knows habits are powerful, good or bad. When we establish an exercise habit—usually a regular schedule of movement activities—it carries us along to our movement activity on those days when we don't really want to do it or when our brain comes up with an unusually large amount of excuses (including the ever clever "I have to wash my hair" excuse). Any slow-starter or avoider knows convincing ourselves to do a movement activity can sometimes be more difficult than the exercise itself.

So how do we get into an exercise habit and get ourselves on the current? Simple. We schedule our exercising.

From the activities in Tip #2, you have a fairly good idea how often and at what time of day you want to move. Combine that with any sports or class schedules from your new exciting movement activities and you can begin to see a schedule forming. Scheduling is good for everyone except those who rebel against anything too structured. For you rebels, it could be helpful to assign days of the week for exercise without any clue what you'll do or when—providing yourselves with loose structure.

ACTIVITY CHOICE: Experiment with scheduling until you find something that works for you. If you rebel against your schedule and stop going, you've probably put too many activities on your list, or too many boring activities on your list. Or you might not enjoy having such a strict schedule.

4. Tell yourself you'll only move for a little bit (in other words, lie). Style: overachiever, slow-starter, avoider

There are some days when our lazy thoughts rule. The excuses are running wild. On those days, there's only one thing stopping us: ourselves. This is when this trick works wonders: we lie to ourselves.

Even when we have habits in place, our lazy brain has a strong power over us. To counteract our lazy thoughts, we can make a promise to our lazy brain that we might not keep. Such a promise might be, "I'll only exercise for fifteen minutes" or it could be "I'll only do my favorite exercises" or "If I workout, I'll buy myself a new dress."

Since our promise is the breakable kind, this trick gives us room. Room to be lazy, but also room for compromise. It buys us time.

Most likely, when we're finally moving, the need to only move for fifteen minutes will disappear. And if it doesn't, no problem. We can keep our promise if we need to, and we've done at least some movement for the day. Any movement, I promise you, is better than nothing.

Another kind of breakable promise you can make is to schedule more exercise knowing you'll probably follow through on 50-75% of it. My younger brother did that when he wanted to get himself to exercise every day. He decided to strive to exercise twice a day. That way, he'd either succeed with his promise or at least get in one workout a day.

See, there are all kinds of way to trick your lazy brain into doing your bidding!

5. Enjoy your activity. Style: All

As I have said before, set yourself up for success. Choose something fun. A friend of mine took strip tease classes. She was highly motivated because she was interested, and she felt good doing it.

6. Be ready. Style: slow-starter, avoider

If you have classes or set times for movement activities, there are some general rules to follow to ensure a great success each time you move.

- Eat two to four hours before your activity and make sure the food is light—I've almost puked and fainted several times from either a too full or too empty stomach and high-intensity sports. Don't let one bad puking experience ruin you for exercise forever. Just know that you reached your limit and don't push yourself so hard the next time. And don't eat what you ate when the incident occurred. For me, drinking coffee close to exercise is a no-no. It makes me really dehydrated. Anything too greasy also makes me sluggish.
- Hydrate—drink water beforehand, during and after.
- Dress in clothes that make you feel good and won't get in your way. Try wicking materials that draw sweat away from your skin and help you feel dry and comfortable. See Tip #8 for more information.

- Brush your teeth—mint has been found to improve performance in movement plus you might feel more comfortable interacting with others knowing you have fresh breath.
- Use deodorant.
- Use whatever works best for you to prevent chafing if that's an issue for you—there are several products on the market for runners and exercisers to lubricate areas normally susceptible to chafing. Or put a Bandaid on that area.
- Bring a towel to wipe off sweat.
- Pull back your hair if you need to.
- If you're heading to the gym or going for a run, have your mp3 player charged and ready with your best motivational playlist. I can't emphasize enough how important music that pumps you up will help you through a workout at the gym!
- Wear supportive shoes.
- Skip the makeup, or wear waterproof makeup—go with what makes you feel most confident.
- Bring a watch if you need it.
- Bring a small snack if you're going to be working out for more than an hour and a half.

When we have all the equipment we need, we feel prepared and more comfortable. This is especially important when we're starting new activities. After the first couple of times, you'll know exactly what you need to bring each time.

7. To Count or Not to Count.

When I was trying to quit smoking in college, I counted every day that I didn't smoke. On the 12th day, it finally hit me that to be a healthy-lunged individual, I'd have to act like one again.

How'd I quit (at least for ten years)?

I stopped counting the days (and drank a lot of coffee).

Counting the days can indicate a punishment perspective. Prisoners count the days of their incarceration, and smokers who try to quit count the days that they haven't smoked. Dieters count the days they've been "good." Counting indicates an abnormal and often painful present moment that must be overcome by sheer will-power, patience and time.

That's why non-smokers don't count cigarette-free days. It's normal to have cigarette-free days. Are you counting the days you exercise? Why are you counting? What are you counting for?

I used to not believe in counting the days I exercised; after all, if you love your exercise activity enough, you don't have to count. You go because you love it.

However, for those who are still struggling to find an exercise activity they love, I do have to admit that counting is a measurable goal, and some people respond really well to numbers. So if you're a numbers/goal person, count away. Just understand that exercise does not have to be punishment.

Recently, I wanted to increase the days I exercised to five a week. I started tracking what I did on my calendar, and it helped me with the initial change to stay consistent. Was it a long-term habit? No. But it was fun for a while.

So, if you're counting, ask yourself why. If it's to motivate you to accomplish a goal, fantastic. If it's because the activity you're doing feels like torture, try a new activity.

8. Dress for Success. Style: Avoider, Slow-Starter

One of my dancer friends brings several outfits to dance class so that she can feel her best while she dances. Try as often as you can to find clothes that you feel beautiful in. I know it can be difficult sometimes—I certainly don't always feel confident in my exercise outfit. But it's important to find clothes that allow you to do what you want to do. If your hair is getting in your eyes, then you need to buy a headband or pull your hair back. You could need looser clothing or tighter clothing.

Here's what I like, just to give you an idea. I like layers. I wear long sleeve shirts until I get warmed up. Underneath I wear a fitted tank top because I don't like sleeves when exercising. I don't like loose t-shirts either because I do activities that require me to be upside down (dance, yoga). In those positions, I'm usually chewing on my t-shirt unless I have something more fitted. Underwear as well is important. If they're too loose, or too tight, I'm always adjusting and not fully comfortable. Honestly, I find traditional-style briefs or bikini briefs are the most comfortable and least likely to ride up.

You'll find as you get started what your personal clothing needs are. It makes a difference. It adds an extra level of comfort and enjoyment to your activity. Never let an uncomfortable outfit prevent you from working out.

Motivated Mover Activities to Try Today or Right Now to Overcome Lazy Brain

---

ACTIVITY CHOICE: Why not go back to the beginning of this chapter and do the activities I recommend if you haven't already? There's no time like the present to overcome your lazy brain and become a motivated mover!

ACTIVITY CHOICE: This is the end of Part 1. Go through the notes you took in Part 1 and fill out the table on the following page. Then continue to Part 2.

What is your exercise style?

What is the time of day you decided to exercise?

Are you working out with people or by yourself?

Are you going to make goals?

Are you going to go to a gym?

What activity did you decide to do? Is it the most exciting and scary one?

Have you gone to your activity yet? If not, write down what day this week you plan on going.

Did you do a walking meditation if you needed extra motivation?

Did you keep an exercise journal? If you didn't, write down what day this week you will begin.

Did you write down your most common excuse and come up with an effective response to make sure you get to your activity?

PART 2

Maintaining Your Momentum

TIP #5

Make Goals, Not Chores

So you've gone through all the tips of getting yourself off the couch and to your fun exercise activity. Now what? How do you keep yourself going long term?

First of all, I commend you for getting this far! If you have not done any exercising yet, go back to the beginning, do the activities in the book, and get to an exercise activity or two before you move on. This book is about gaining motivation and keeping motivation to exercise. So don't wait. Go do it. Start now.

Let's assume you're getting to the gym or going to your activity because you enjoy it. You're having fun. You're ignoring your lazy brain and getting there fairly consistently.

You might be wondering by now...shouldn't I have a goal?

Yes...and no....

Here's what I mean. The only reason we would want to be cautious about setting goals is that, if we're not careful, we can make what could be a very joyful and fun experience into a totally lame chore. Then exercise becomes a "Should," (as I mentioned several times throughout this book) and suddenly it's even more difficult to motivate ourselves.

So this chapter is here to help you figure out which goals help you and which ones hinder you.

When Goals Miss the Mark

Sometimes the goals you thought were so awesome on New Year's Eve when you had one too many glasses of wine just don't seem as fun when you actually have to do them.

Read on to see if these examples resonate with you:

GOALS THAT IGNORE WHAT OUR BODIES CAN OR CAN'T DO: Let's take an example of my good friend, Sarah, a classic achiever. When stress was affecting her health, she set a goal to wake up every day at 5am to run. Of course, she attacked her goal with the confidence of someone who knows she's going to accomplish her goal. She continued running even though her knees really hurt because she could see some cardio and de-stressing benefit from it. But the pain got worse. Eventually, her knees gave her so much trouble she had to stop running completely.

GOALS OUT OF OUR FITNESS ZONE: Think about my friend who signed up for a gym membership with a goal to lose weight and only went twice. She pushed herself so hard that she felt terrible, puked and then didn't go back for years.

GOALS THAT REQUIRE COMPLETE COMMITMENT AND DON'T INCORPORATE REAL LIFE: Another friend of mine did a program and was solidly consistent for six weeks. Then she got the flu. Two weeks later, she had abandoned her goal completely.

Sound familiar?

The problem for most of us is not that we have trouble *beginning our goals* (though for some of us, even beginning is hard), the problem is *continuing* with it. And that's because we started with the *wrong goal* and chose the *wrong approach* in accomplishing it.

When we start with the wrong goal, we get the wrong result.

What are the Wrong Goals?

Wrong goals are objectives that don't support us physically, mentally and spiritually. Examples of unsupportive goals include the following: promising to go to the gym five times a week when we hate the gym, swearing we'll swim laps three times a week when putting our head under water makes us panicky, or pushing ourselves to attend dance classes every week when we know we're not inspired by dancing.

What are Wrong Approaches?

Any form of the "Do or Die" approach is a wrong approach: continuing to exercise when it hurts our knees or other joints in a very acute way, or when we refuse to modify movement to make it possible for us to complete the exercise.

I'm using "us" here because I can be a "Do or Die" woman, too. It's hard to admit when I feel faint or nauseous or when my high-arched feet hurt. It feels a lot like failure.

"I'm going to do this, even if it kills me" is the approach I'd like you to eliminate.

There's an easier, gentler way. Exercise doesn't have to be such a struggle.

What is the Right Approach?

When considering the right approach, all I ask is one simple thing: **make it fun**. You can't treat exercise like a chore. Well, technically, you can. But why would you want to?

It's a common misconception that movement activities should only be hard work and pain. Movement activities can be hard work and cause muscle soreness, but they can also be the time of your life!

Think of it like this: "I'm going to do this, see if my body can handle it, and if it can, I'm going to continue because I'm having fun!"

What are the Right Goals?

Goals are very personal, so the goal that might make me so excited (say, a goal to attend salsa class on Thursdays consistently and trampoline aerobics on Tuesday), might make your hair stand up on end in horror at how WRONG that goal is for you.

Where I *can* guide you is in telling you the right goal for you is simply the one that makes you happy and excited.

There are many resources out there offering advice about how to set goals. For example, the National Academy of Sports Medicine

(NASM) says your goals need to be the following if you're going to accomplish them:

- **Specific**

  Pick a clear goal. One where you can easily imagine the end-result. For example, running a mile without stopping is a much clearer goal than "getting healthy."

- **Challenging**

  Goals that are too easy lead to boredom. The exciting goals are ones that are difficult enough to push you to grow in some way. They will help you discover what you're capable of. For example, setting a goal to run/walk a 5k might be an appropriately challenging goal if you've started walking recently.

- **Approaching**

  Your goals need to be phrased in a positive manner. Avoid negative words. For example, instead of saying, "I'm not going to stop exercising like I did last year," you can put it positively, "I will exercise every other day for at least 30 minutes."

- **Measurable**

  Nebulous goals are less effective because we can't tell when we've accomplished them. Something exact involving numbers is recommended. For example, the immeasurable but nice goal of wanting to "get fit" could be switched to "I want to walk a mile in under 40 minutes."

- **Proximal (soon)**

  Your goals should be small enough so you can accomplish them in the near future. Small, quick wins are more motivating than a year-long struggle...though after many quick wins, training for something long-term like marathons might become very doable for you. For example, "It is July 1st. I want to be able to do 5 push-ups on my knees by the end of July."

- **Inspirational**

  Your goals should make you excited! For example, "I want to run a 10k for that charity" or "I've always wanted to bike up that hill..."

An example of a NASM-approved goal would be: *I want to be able to run/walk a half marathon without injury within six months of training.* The smaller goal might be: *I want to run/walk a 5k within three month of training.* It's a measurable, very specific goal. It's phrased with positive language. It's challenging—but not impossible—and it has a relatively close due date, and depending on who you are, it might inspire you.

The Best Kind of Goal is Goals

I think people in the fitness industry gloss over the most important part of goal-setting, and the one I have difficulty with. It's adding an "s" to goal and making it goals. Say we have a goal, and we accomplish it. What then?

If we don't set new goals while we're within reach of our first goal, we're more likely to quit once it's accomplished, negating all our hard work. If we use the previous example of the NASM-approved goal, we might add a new goal as we approached our half marathon goal to do a marathon in another six months of training.

Lofty Dreams into Realizable Goals

What have you always wanted to accomplish with fitness? Shoot a goal in soccer? Perform downward dog in yoga? Dance in a dance show? Hike to the top of a mountain?

I heard a friend of a friend say she wanted to be a super yoga girl. What does that mean to her? For this exercise, she could translate this dream into something more measurable, like "I'd like to go to yoga four times a week for a month." Her follow-up goal might be to go to yoga four times a week for four months total. Once she's in class, she most likely will discover new goals she'd like to accomplish as well.

ACTIVITY CHOICE: Write your dreams down and translate them into the measurable and specific goals that excite and inspire you. Make sure you write down follow-up goals that will keep you going. Remember, determination and discipline are incredible forces, but they won't count if the exercise you do isn't any fun or doesn't give you any pleasure. So make sure it's fun!

Write down your dreams and the translation to measurable goals in your notebook right now if you'd like.

1. What is your exercise **dream**?
2. What is the translation to your exercise **goal**?
3. What are some possible **follow-up goals**?

Do you have your goals? Are you excited about them? You're going to keep your body in mind when you start to accomplish them, right?

Goals and a Single Purpose

With all that said, there is the other side of goals. I commend you if you can sustain moving the bar higher and higher for your whole life. Some people excel with goals. Others get burnt out with that method, and ask, "When will enough be enough?"

Think about how you can sustain your exercise motivation throughout your life. Is it with goals? Is it with the quality of your movement activity? A combination?

Constantly striving to achieve goals can be difficult. That's why I recommend having an overall purpose to your fitness—an umbrella statement that will help you when all else fails. Something that guides you every day, goal or no goal. I highly encourage you to adopt this purpose so you live a long and joyful life. Are you ready? Drum roll, please...

Motivated Mover Purpose
"I will focus on fun when I exercise in some way,
shape or form almost every day."

Throughout my workout history, I've had times when I have been very focused on accomplishing fitness goals. During other times (especially in the last year), I relied on my umbrella purpose.

Having both goals and a purpose can motivate you through the good times and buoy you through the bad times.

The Skinny on Our Exercise Goal

Most women want to be thinner than they are right now. It's not surprising considering the buzz in the media about obesity and messages we receive daily that "thin is in." Ugh, don't get me started, ladies!

I can't prevent you from wanting to lose weight, but this book is about exercising for fun and enjoying the feeling of your body moving. Sometimes that can be inconsistent with a punishment/weight-loss perspective. Try shelving your weight loss goals and try on this method for a while. The motivated mover purpose is a helpful perspective for making exercise a **permanent part of your life**, not just a temporary fix.

I was reading an article by Dr. Shawn Henry, an assistant professor with Pacific University's Exercise Science department, and I really liked what he said about the goal of a fitness program—it was not to lose weight so much as to enhance the quality of life. That's what we're shooting for here, too. You can improve your quality of life **without the difficult prerequisite of hitting a certain weight or BMI number.**

Goals, I have found at least for me, are fragile. With the slightest interruption, goals can often derail completely. Having goals plus the purpose can push you past inertia. It keeps you returning to exercise, not because you have to but because you want to.

Motivated Mover Activities to Try Today or Right Now to Choose Goals

---

ACTIVITY CHOICE: Think about some of your fitness dreams. You might have a lot of body image dreams for now. Set aside the image goals for now. Then allow yourself to think of what kind of performance goals you want to accomplish: Run a mile without stopping? Climb a mountain? Bike to your work? Use the activity in the chapter to translate your dreams into measurable goals. Put them on your schedule and get started! If you get frustrated, no worries, remember your umbrella purpose to shield you from the "rain."

ACTIVITY CHOICE: Write down the motivated mover purpose and place it where you'll be reminded to exercise!

TIP #6

If Life Gives You Hills, Learn to Shift Gears:

Cultivating Lifelong Enthusiasm

Wow! We've done a lot. We've meditated, thought of fun movement activities (and actually did them), and figured out practical ways to overcome lazy brain. We've set some goals to keep us going and have our purpose for times when our goals don't pan out.

In this chapter, we will work on honing our lifelong enthusiasm.

How to Shift to Your Lifelong Enthusiasm

I believe we have two very different qualities of enthusiasm on which to rely. One is short-term enthusiasm, the other lifelong. **We need both** if we want to stay motivated to exercise. A good example of the short-term kind is the excitement we feel when we first start a fitness program. Our hopes are high, the highest even! We have a lot of passion. We can't wait to get started.

Short-term enthusiasm is like fifth gear in a car: great for high speeds, not great for power. We discover this when, after six weeks of intensive exercising later, our short-term enthusiasm has diminished significantly. If we don't learn to shift gears to a different type of enthusiasm, we will have trouble keeping our goals. We will stall out.

Life can often trigger the demise of short-term enthusiasm: We get sick or injured. Someone in our family is ill. Work gets extremely busy. We get a bout of insomnia. We stop exercising for two weeks. When we attempt to start again, the enthusiasm we had six weeks ago is gone.

Short-term enthusiasm is always founded on a vision of the future. We will be skinnier. We will be happier. The hills of life are reality checks: what we thought would only take six weeks will take much longer. We are disappointed. That disappointment snuffs out our short-term enthusiasm for exercise.

So how do we learn to shift to our lifelong enthusiasm? What does that transformation look like? Does our thinking change?

Lifelong enthusiasm is founded on past and present results rather than a vision of the future. To shift gears to lifelong enthusiasm we have to focus on those benefits that *have happened* already and *are happening* currently. Transformation and future happiness will come, but in their own due time. And if you look closely enough, they are happening right now. We must let go of our imagined future selves and learn to enjoy the feeling of moving in the bodies we have right now.

ACTIVITY CHOICE: With no pressure and no worry about future results, you're free to choose the movement activity you love. If you feel you're operating with short-term enthusiasm, imagine there is no tomorrow. Given only this day and the mission to go move your body, which movement activity would you choose to do? Write a few ideas in your notebook.

Begin to notice which movement activities you enjoy in the moment of doing them. Find new movement activities to complement the ones you already enjoy. If you already go to the gym, take some classes on your off-days, or add a sport.

Use the exercise journal in Tip #3 to help you if you have trouble paying attention to your body and how your body and mind feel during and after your activity.

To Shift to Lifelong Enthusiasm, Go at <u>Your Own Pace</u>

In the familiar fable *The Tortoise and the Hare*, the tortoise and the hare decide to race each other. The hare is so confident she'll win, she decides to take a nap halfway through the race. The tortoise, who started off much slower than the hare, continues on, slow and steady. Lo and behold, while the hare naps, the tortoise wins the race.

Another part of lifelong enthusiasm is embracing the times when you are the hare, quick and lithe, and when you are the tortoise, slow and plodding. You might try a new fitness activity and be the best at it quickly. If that's you, great.

Most likely though, if you're starting a new exercise activity, you might relate more to the tortoise. It can be difficult to start a new activity and watch everyone else excel at it, while you flail about. Imagine what it must've been like for the tortoise to watch the back of the hare recede into the distance. But look what happened in the end. The tortoise found success, too. And so will you. Remember, everyone has a beginning phase. And after a lot of practice, they move better and better.

In case you just can't relate to a bunch of animals, check out Cliff Young, a farmer from Australia who decided to compete in a 5-day ultra-marathon. When the race began, he was the slowest. He shuffled while others ran long strides. His competitors left him in the dust. But after several days, he had passed his strongest competitors. What happened? While the runners stopped to sleep each night, Cliff kept going. And just like the tortoise, he won.

My friend Lua told me a great metaphor for beginning exercise. "Our training sessions are like this book," she said and held up a 300-page book. "Each time we train," she said and opened the book, "it's one page read in this book." She flipped over one page. "With one training session, you haven't made much of a dent in the book. But after 30 or 40 training sessions," she said and flipped over a chunk of the book, "you can start to see that you've made progress."

I loved this metaphor because it's true. After 200 sessions of your movement activity, your body will feel different. Your mind will feel changed, too. I went to approximately 200-240 Sunday dance classes/rehearsals over five years (and I counted them up right now to tell you, not because I was counting along the way). I can attest it's true. My body and ability were far different after five years than when I first started the class.

I had to relearn my own advice and accept that I'm still, most of the time, a tortoise when I begin an activity. When I lived in Santiago, Chile, I bought a bike to get around the city. I love bicycling and wanted to bike to the top of a local hill called Cerro San Cristobal.

I did not accept being a tortoise easily. I hated that all the other cyclists were faster than me. Even the runners were passing me! How embarrassing!

When I tried to push myself to go faster than my beginner pace, I made myself sick. I had to accept that I was not the hare but the tortoise in that moment. Going my pace made biking fun, and I was more willing to go consistently because of it. Go your pace so you can enjoy the moment and let the lifelong enthusiasm in you blossom.

Shift to Lifelong Enthusiasm by Acknowledging You Might Be in the Pre-Beginning Phase

Sometimes, when you start a new movement activity, your beginning is pre-beginning and you can't do the movement as the instructor does it. There's preschool before kindergarten.

Why not give yourself a pre-exercise environment and modify the movement to what you can do? Do you need to do the movement in a chair? Or work your legs and forget about your arms? Can't do a push up? Try it against a wall. Do the movement that you can maintain. Maybe it's just walking in place while others run. Listen to what your body is telling you, and let it guide you.

In my dance class and yoga class, we often talk about not knowing what body we'll be bringing to class. Our body moves differently day to day. If we haven't danced in a while, our muscles feel tight or less responsive. If we haven't had enough sleep, we might be slower.

When we go at our own pace, we will be much happier to pay attention to our bodies because they won't be crying out for us to stop (well, not as loudly anyway). The easiest way to shift to your lifelong enthusiasm once your short-term enthusiasm wanes is to pay attention to present sensations (wow! I'm not breathing as hard at the top of the stairs!).

Lifelong Enthusiasm is Fostered with a Light Grip, Not a Vice Grip!

Another aspect of lifelong enthusiasm is in letting go of all-or-nothing restrictive thinking. Think of your mind as a cat. It does what it wants most of the time. Just like a cat, if you restrict your mind and squeeze too tight, it will struggle to be free. For the short term, you can hold onto it. But in the long run, you have to let it go or risk injury.

But similarly, if you make something inviting—like a blanket on a warm bed—your cat will happily curl up and begin to purr. If we can make exercise enjoyable, our minds will also begin to purr.

The biggest vice grip we have on our minds and bodies is the all-or-nothing mentality. We often have all-or-nothing thinking when it comes to diet and fitness programs, especially those promising significant weight loss. We either follow the program closely using short-term enthusiasm and restriction to drive us (and then we eventually give it up) or we don't do it at all.

Personally, I dislike diets. Calorie counting and restrictions are not fun, and I don't think they work long term. My issue with diets—besides not having enough energy to feel strong when I exercise—is that food restrictions make certain foods seem more special or rare, foods I would eat in moderation (and with pleasure) without a diet; and when they're rare, I crave them more. With strong cravings, my ability to resist is diminished. Voila—I've abandoned my diet completely and pigged out on the food I've been missing.

It's happened to many of us. A great example of this was with a friend of mine. My friend was trying a low-carb diet. One of the restrictions was she wasn't allowed to eat potatoes. So of course, she couldn't stop thinking about them. The funny part is she never craved potatoes normally! She didn't even like them much. It was just the thought of not being able to have them—the restriction—that made potatoes a rarity and then a craving.

Programs put too many restrictions on us. When we fail at one restriction, we often decide we've failed at all of them (which is not true).

It happened to a client of mine. A month into personal training, a client with that all-or-nothing mentality didn't show up for training. She didn't show up for several weeks. Eventually, she returned and explained what had happened.

She had eaten a lot of fast food the first week. Her assumption was that since she'd failed at meeting all of her dietary requirements she had set for herself, she had failed at everything fitness, including exercise. So she stopped coming to the gym for personal training, too. Her thinking was: "Why keep going when I've already failed?" Sound familiar?

But I understand. There's a lot of fear there, too. Disappointment and fear. Fear that if we try again, we will fail again. Or that we won't be able to perform what is asked of us. It's difficult to overcome those fears and continue on.

Marilyn Wann, author of *Fat!So?*, said it best in an interview for a blog I started a few years ago: "If you come at fitness and good nutrition as a form of punishment for a bad body, it just won't last. Humans can only willingly do a form of punishment for about five or six weeks. Eating less and exercising more are wonderful behaviors. But attaching those behaviors to a 'poison pill' [weight-loss goal] doesn't work."

To start a new exercise habit, we WILL need to squeeze our minds a little. We will need to push ourselves at least a little to exercise. So we need to learn where we can squeeze a lot and where squeezing a lot will result in our complete refusal to exercise at all.

Here's what I suggest for avoiding a rebellion and losing your lifelong enthusiasm:

1. Follow this book and find exercises that are fun and/or make you feel good. This will help you feel more free from restrictions and motivate you in a positive manner instead of in a restrictive manner.

2. Make sure you eat a few hours before you exercise. Many of you might try to accompany a food restriction with the motivated mover method. I am saying to you right now, eat. Please. You have to be having fun as a motivated mover, and nothing's fun about trying to get your body to move a lot when you're hungry.

Shifting to Lifelong Enthusiasm will Promote Consistency and Harmony

Part of the definition of "consistency" in the Merriam-Webster dictionary is that it is marked by harmony, regularity or steady continuity. When we're on a restrictive program, we aren't in harmony with our mind. Our cat-mind is already squirming and struggling to get free. But it can be in harmony with an activity of your choosing that you find enjoyable. It can be in agreement with food that your body likes—you know, the kind of food that makes you feel energetic and light after eating it?

The more you have lifelong enthusiasm, the more consistent you will become. Cultivate lifelong enthusiasm through the following (some of which we discussed in earlier tips):

- **A flexible mentality that is opposite of the all-or-nothing attitude**: remember, life always throws challenges your way. There will be days you can't exercise. But it's with that flexible "I'll continue where I left off" mentality that makes exercise a consistent part of your life.
- **Fun, varied activities:** when it's fun, you'll go more often. The easiest way to stay on course is to like the course you're on.
- **Activities at your physical fitness level that challenge but don't fatigue you:** choose activities and modify them to your current exercise level. If you can't do a push-up on the ground, feeling bad is not the answer. Do push-ups on the wall first. This helps you from getting discouraged.
- **Properly fueling your body before exercise:** you'll feel so good when you find the food that makes exercise easier and fun.
- **Charged up Qi, or a feeling that powers you and gives you energy:** life can still be tough and challenging, you may still feel sad, but when you can, boost your Qi through meditation to make getting to exercise easier.
- **Strong, motivating personal reasons for showing up to your movement activities:** what can exercise do for

you? Does it clear your head? Make you happier? Help you sleep? Balance your energy?

Motivated Mover Activities to Try Today or Right Now to Shift to Your Lifelong Enthusiasm

---

ACTIVITY CHOICE: Simple. Go back and do the activity at the beginning of this chapter. If you haven't yet done the activities in previous chapters, why not try them today?

ACTIVITY CHOICE: Pay attention to how you feel after you exercise. Are you happier? Use your exercise journal. When it's time to go exercise each day, remind yourself of the results you *already feel* to cultivate your lifelong enthusiasm.

ACTIVITY CHOICE: A lifetime can be overwhelming to think about. Why not commit to trying your exercise activity of choice for three months? Why not shelve your idea to do an all-or-nothing program until you see how well you do with the tips in this book?

TIP #7

You Can Do It!

Becoming Your Own Sports Psychologist

What do you tell yourself about your self-worth, the value of your body before you exercise? What do you tell yourself when you're exercising?

Negative self-talk can hinder your movement motivation. It saps your mental energy and your internal joy. It's more difficult to do movement activities when you're telling yourself you look ugly in the outfit you have on or that you're so much fatter than everyone else there or that you can't do it. Imagine you had a personal trainer or coach guiding you. How well would you perform if they were telling you, "You'll never get it! You're the worst I've ever seen! What made you decide to even try this?"

My guess is not very well.

Whatever movement activity you choose will at some point challenge you. It might already be challenging. Or as you advance, you'll find it more and more difficult. And at that point, how you think will determine how you perform. A part of any activity is mental.

Imagination and thoughts are powerful—they trigger your nervous system. Think about it. You have physical sensations like butterflies in your stomach when you're nervous or a heavy feeling in your shoulders if you're sad. Conversely, you can create good physical sensations with positive thoughts and images. Several studies confirm the power of imagination. They show that our nervous system is activated in similar ways, regardless of whether we're imagining doing an activity or actually performing it.

I tested this when understudying for the Linda Bair Modern Dance Company. Every week we'd learn new choreography, a movement vocabulary that felt awkward to me. Every evening, when I drove home, washed dishes, or had a free moment, I imagined myself doing the new choreography in my head. My movement improved, and I became known for having a great memory for movement.

A psychologist named Milton H. Erickson trained himself to walk after being paralyzed by polio by imagining himself walking and repeating the memories of how moving felt.

Knowing how thoughts can affect movement both positively and negatively, it is imperative we cut negative thinking as much as possible. We're going to practice being our own sports psychologists here.

Sports psychologists work with athletes to improve their performance by helping them manage their emotions and thoughts. So if we use the techniques a sports psychologist uses, we can train our nervous system to perform more effectively and move with greater ease.

What techniques will we use? Sports psychologists have several techniques they use in their work with athletes, including visualization, positive self-talk, relaxation, focus and confidence building. We're going to practice some of these techniques here.

Visualization

If visualization can help elite athletes, surely it can help us, too—even with a task as simple as psyching ourselves up for exercise. Every day you plan to exercise, take a moment in the morning to imagine yourself driving to your activity and having fun during the activity. Imagine the feeling of well-being in your body and mind after you have accomplished your activity. The feeling part is important.

Visualization is more than using your vision. Utilize your imagination and activate all your senses. What sounds do you imagine? What do you smell? Breathe deeply. Sit with those good feelings for a minute or two before starting your day. These visualizations can be seeds you plant that grow throughout the day and make you more motivated to exercise.

You can also use visualization for review. If you're taking a class, you can review the movement you learned in your head. The great thing about imagination is you can use it anywhere (obviously!), especially in those time when your mind isn't occupied—sitting in traffic, brushing your teeth, washing dishes, or standing in line.

Positive Self-Talk

Telling yourself "yes I can" is one of the best ways to counteract any negative thoughts coming to your mind. A simple "I can do it. I know I can!" when your activity pushes you can make the difference between continuing and quitting.

When an athlete is consistently being bested by the competition, the reason is often not that they lack skill but that they have limiting beliefs about their capabilities. You don't even notice you have limiting beliefs. But they're there. They appear when you avoid certain exercises because you assume you couldn't possibly do them, when you really don't know yet.

You can also use affirmations, like "I am an athlete" or "I am capable of finishing this race" to drown out the negative self-talk.

I used to use this technique in personal training. If my clients were struggling, I would tell them, "Tell yourself, 'Yes, I can finish this. I can.' I would usually see a slight energy come back in their eyes, and their next few reps would have more power and energy. Just by three words. "Yes I can."

Try it for yourself.

Relaxation

Rellllllaaaaxxxxxxx. Easier said than done. But if you experience a lot of tension before going to exercise—are you nervous or worried about how you'll do?—try progressive relaxation.

With progressive relaxation, you tense and relax specific muscle groups. Tense and relax your feet and calves. Tense and relax your thighs. Tense and relax your stomach. Go through your whole body tensing and relaxing. You might discover certain areas of the body are already tense, like your neck or shoulders or facial muscles.

Realizing that your muscle is already tense can help you relax areas more completely.

Practicing Focus

Studies show athletic performance is enhanced by mindfulness and acceptance of present circumstances. Becoming aware and focused on your physical state is called associative body monitoring. This has helped many athletes.

Basically, pay attention to your body. Focus on your breathing. Focus on muscles tensed unnecessarily. Are your facial muscles tense? Shoulders? How are you feeling? Do you feel good? Fatigued? By paying attention to physical sensations, you can better understand how your body reacts to challenges.

Building Confidence

Do it again.

One of the best ways to build your confidence is to repeat your activity. Practice is the key to improvement with your activity. When you accomplish your goal, whatever it may be, repeat it before moving on to a new goal. Master it so you can't write it off as luck.

The Virtuous Cycle

Exercise makes your mind and heart and soul feel good! Your mood is lifted, which changes your self-talk from negative to more and more positive. It's that fantastic virtuous cycle I talked about in Tip #3. The more you move, the more you'll feel good and energetic, the more you'll feel like moving, the more you'll feel good and energetic, and so on. It's no wonder exercise is used as a part of treatment for clinical depression and anxiety. Studies show exercise can improve your body-image esteem and decrease those negative feelings like confusion, sadness, anger and tension. One study pointed to yoga as promising for promoting well-being in depressed patients. There's even some evidence that links exercise with improved brain function in older adults.

Motivated Mover Activities to Try Today or Right
Now to Become Your Own Sports Psychologist

ACTIVITY CHOICE: Knowledge is only potential power. We can listen to all this information and say, "yes, that sounds right," but nothing beats action and experience—our potential power put into motion. So, take one of the sports psychology suggestions (visualization, relaxation, focus) and apply it to the exercise activity you're going to do today.

TIP #8

Conquer the Details: Guides to Exercising at Home or at the Gym

This wouldn't be much of a book if I didn't at least touch on the practical details of setting out to exercise. If you've followed along in the book, you've already begun moving. If you still need a little boost, or are getting stuck and overwhelmed with the small details of exercise, then this chapter is for you!

I can't cover every activity of course, but I can help you get started. For a complete list of recommended books to help you continue your movement journey, see Appendix II.

Exercise at Home Guide

PROS: convenience, comfortable (no one's watching)

CONS: home distractions prevent exercise, lack of variety (videos), lack of challenge

I commend anyone who can work out consistently at home. You all deserve a huge pat on the back. I consider consistent home workouts the MOST difficult to perform.

Why? I think of home as a place of rest, relaxation and safety. I don't yearn to get home to sweat. Plus I get distracted at home. There are too many soft places to rest, too many other activities that seem like more fun.

But of course, sometimes circumstances make it necessary for you to work out at home. Money, injury, small children, convenience, bad weather outside, general laziness—can all conspire to make a home workout your best option.

Keep the following tips in mind for home exercising:

- Those just beginning exercise might benefit from starting with an exercise video that guides you through all the steps. Look for ones that offer you beginner, intermediate and advanced modifications. You can go to the library to rent DVDs or go online to YouTube to get free ones. Press play, and off you go!

- If you hate aerobics programs because of the peppy instructors, there are plenty of more edgy, hard-core workout programs. A very popular workout is Power 90X. Any other video that contains the word Boot Camp should be more edgy. I also recommend the Hip Hop Island Girl video for a different type of fun workout.

- Once you have established a consistent routine (and know you WILL continue to work out at home), consider buying an interactive video game console for a combination of exercise and games.
- Spice up your video variety, too, by checking out yoga, Pilates and Tai Chi fitness videos.
- You can also put on some rockin' music and dance. If you like goals, set an amount of time you'll dance for.
- After becoming more familiar with your body and how it moves, create your own exercise routine using body weight exercises. See below for a sample 30-minute workout. If you don't know how to do these exercises, a quick look on the Internet can give you videos on how to perform each one.

Sample Home Body-Weight Routine
Beginner/Intermediate

Exercise	# of reps or duration	Muscles
☐ High knees/marching	1 minute	aerobic warm up
☐ Jumping jacks	1 minute	aerobic warm up
☐ Plank	15 to 30 seconds hold, 2x	arms, abdominal
☐ Roman Deadlift	10 reps	butt, legs, calves, back
☐ Push-ups (wall, knees, full)	10 reps	arms, chest, back
☐ Sit-up Twists	10 reps	abdominal, back
☐ Step-up overhead press with balance	10 reps per leg	total body and balance

Use .5 liter or 1 liter plastic bottles filled with water for weights if you don't have dumbbells available. Tempo for each is as follows: lift the weight for 1 second, hold 2 seconds, lower for 4 seconds (sit-up twists, step-up overhead press). Sometimes exercises start with the lowering element, and then it would be reversed: Lower for 4 seconds, hold for 2 seconds, lift back up for 1 second (push-ups, roman deadlift). Don't worry about tempo if it seems too complicated. Do your best.

If you cannot lift the required number of repetitions, the exercise is too advanced for you. Modify it by reducing the pounds of the weights, not using weights, reducing the time or reducing the angle of your body. For example, if push-ups on the knees is too difficult, try push-ups against the wall or a counter—with an easier angle of incline.

Remember to breathe.

After mastering this routine, switch it up with new exercises you can find online. When designing a routine, there are really an incredible amount of options. For a beginner, design routines that challenge the whole body and incorporate a balance element to train your nervous system, too.

An easy way to design your own is to start with the top of your body and work your way down. Find exercises for each of the following muscle groups: shoulders, back, chest, arms, abdominal muscles (stomach), butt, and upper and lower legs. Search for exercises for each muscle group. If you're still at a loss for where to begin, and the Internet and books don't seem to work for you, hire a personal trainer that comes to homes to guide you through exercises. After a while, you'll begin to see how to put exercise routines together.

You may find you can't do the exercises on the video yet or can only do a portion of a routine. If you can, great! Do what you can and praise yourself often for what you do accomplish. If getting yourself out of bed or out of your chair is an accomplishment, pat yourself on the back. If walking to the street corner and back is what you can do, great! Some of these home exercise suggestions can be modified by sitting in a chair if it's difficult for you to stand. For example, you can do videos or dancing while in a chair.

We all have a place from which we start. Be proud that you have begun, where ever that beginning place is.

What Equipment You Need for Home Exercising

You really only need comfortable clothes that don't chafe or bind and shoes that feel good on your feet. And some people even go without shoes.

If you want to do more complex home routines, I recommend:

- Foam roller (SMR)—to correct posture and reduce soreness (I mentioned the foam roller in Tip #4)
- Yoga mat—exercises feel better on a mat instead of a rug
- Stability ball—challenge your muscles, balance and nervous system

- Tubes and bands—alternatives to weights
- Medicine ball—weighted ball used in exercises designed to increase your power (force and strength)
- Weights—an investment for those who know they're going to be consistent with it

Good luck with your home workouts! If you discover you're not consistently exercising, it's time to go search for a gym that fits you.

Gym Guide

PROS: gets you out of the house, easier to establish habits, fewer interruptions, social, lots of equipment, classes, personal trainers, convenience

CONS: intimidating, boring, sometimes it's an aggressive atmosphere

Here are the best tips I can give those of you who are beginners to the gym scene:

- Choose an attitude. I always feel more comfortable pretending like I own the gym and have worked out every day there for years. Others feel really comfortable being goofy and admitting they have no idea what they're doing. Go with what works for you. At the very least, remind yourself that you have *every right to be there!*

- See if the gym offers a free orientation session with a personal trainer—this can help you become more comfortable with the gym and its equipment
- Go with a friend who can show you the ropes and help you feel comfy
- Bring a towel (for wiping your sweat off the equipment— ewww I know!), water bottle, hair pulled back and out of your face (or a ball cap works too), and pen and paper if you're going to record your weight lifting.
- If you don't like watching TV during your cardio workout, bring a book or magazine, and/or an mp3 player to entertain you.
- Wipe down cardio equipment with the disinfectant spray and towel provided by the gym before and after your workout.
- If you're open to forming friendships, leave your music at home and start up a conversation. If you're not, use closed body language. Send the "I'm totally unapproachable" signal if you don't want to chat with anyone. Wear a hat. Wear headphones. This combo will prevent most people from approaching you, ensuring you a private workout in a crowded gym.
- Manage your sweat: wear wicking clothes, deodorant, comfortable socks, bring a towel.
- Ignore the people who might stare at you blankly. They're

not really staring at you but are mired in their own "stuff" like what's happening at work, how much they're suffering in their workout from exhaustion or boredom, or running through a fight they had with a spouse. If they are staring at you, so what? You're staring at them, right?

- Use equipment freely and slowly. Read directions if it's the first time using it. Take time to adjust weights to exactly what feels comfortable. Don't rush. Set up equipment to match your pivot points (knees and elbows and hips). If you have trouble adjusting something, ask someone for help or move on to another machine. If you are large, talk to the gym before signing up to find out what the machines' weight limitations are. If you're too heavy or big for machines, lift with the free weights or cables instead.

- Allow someone to "work in" if they so wish. This means that once you finish your set, the other person will hop onto the machine for their set. You'll alternate. Don't be upset if when you ask to work in with someone they ask you to wait—most likely they're on their last set and would rather just finish it out.

- The peak times at most gyms are M-Th 5:30am-7:30am; 5:30pm-7:30pm. Go there at those times if you're okay with lots of people. Choose another time if you're not.

- Don't pay more than $25-$75 per month per membership. See if your job offers a discount for a gym membership before signing anything. Don't do anything except a month-to-month contract. Especially if you're starting out, entering into a 2-year contract without knowing whether you'll consistently attend is not a good idea. Plus, independent gyms can go bankrupt and leave you without your money or a gym.

- Make the gym convenient for you. I normally go to a gym near my job so I can drive right over without going home first. For me, going home is the exercise kiss of death. Home is curling up on the softest couch in the world with a novel in hand and a cup of tea. Once I arrive, I'm in for the night.
- Familiarize yourself with strength training terms like:
  - Reps or repetitions—number of times you perform the action of lifting and coming back to start
  - Set—a group of repetitions
  - Tempo—the pace with which you perform each repetition

To learn how to design a workout for yourself at the gym, take a look at the exercises I suggested in the Home Guide. The same applies here. You'll just have more options for weights and exercises at the gym.

What to Look for in a Gym

Finding the right gym is like finding a good company to work for, or finding a good partner. It helps if you know what you're looking for. And to know what you're looking for, you have to know a little bit about gym preferences. Luckily for us, we've been working on ourselves for a good portion of this book and should have a fairly good idea about ourselves by now.

For example, I know I'm lazy so I need to have a location five minutes away from home or work or both. I like small environments because I'm shy, and it's easier to get to know people when there are fewer of them around. It also means I hate an aggressive sales pitch. I have no kids so a family environment isn't necessary. I like a lot of variety, so a gym with a pool and/or racquetball courts is fun but not a necessity.

To help you with your search, I've outlined some items to think about:

Gym Search Worksheet

ACTIVITY CHOICE: Put a check next to the most important features of a gym.

	Gym Feature	What It Could Mean to You
☐	Location close to work	Working out right before or right after work
☐	Location close to home	Working out on weekends is easy
☐	Multiple locations	You can still workout when you travel (yay!)
☐	Indoor Lap Pool	You can swim even through harsh winters
☐	Outdoor Lap Pool	You won't have to smell that chlorine smell as much as in an indoor pool

☐	Kid's Pool	Family environment
☐	Brand New Equipment	Machines might be better equipped to match a variety of body sizes (older equipment was designed for men)
☐	Well-Maintained Equipment	No sticking weights or loose parts
☐	Many Elliptical Machines	If you have bad knees, elliptical machines can reduce stress on your joints while you exercise
☐	Lots of People	Social
☐	Few People	No waiting
☐	Televisions	To pass the time quicker
☐	No televisions	Rather listen to music
☐	Basketball Court	Variety of movement activities; opportunity to reacquaint yourself with this sport
☐	Basketball League	You have the potential to join a team
☐	Racquetball Court	Variety of movement activities; opportunity to reacquaint yourself with this sport
☐	Tennis Court	Variety of movement activities; opportunity to reacquaint yourself with this sport
☐	Tennis League	You have the potential to join a team
☐	Stretching Area	You won't be crowded when stretching or doing abdominal exercises
☐	Aerobic Room	Variety of movement activities with classes

☐	Month-to-Month Membership	You'll have the flexibility to cancel or freeze the membership if you realize you're not using it
☐	Friendly Staff	To field questions, help with equipment or introduce you to other exercisers
☐	Mellow Atmosphere	Some places cater to a large variety of people, all sizes and ages.
☐	High-energy Atmosphere	Some places cater to bodybuilders and attract more singles. If you fit into that category and enjoy the vibe, going to the gym might be as fun as going to a club.
☐	Daycare	Family Environment
☐	Ample Parking	Well-lit at night and easy to park
☐	Quick Drive	No traffic, convenient
☐	No Aggressive Sales Pitch	Want to make a decision without pressure

ACTIVITY CHOICE: Now write your top five priorities in your notebook.

Make sure your gym meets these requirements before signing up. Don't give up until you find one that's right for you. One of my favorites is the YMCA: the one I know of has basketball and racquetball courts, two pools, a free weights room, a machines room, and a cardio room. The machines also have a computer program that monitors how much you lift so you don't have to bring anything with you.

My other favorite gym was a hole-in-the-wall place in Santiago (lot of good that does for you in the States, I know). I thought I wouldn't like the small independent gym, but as it turns out, although it didn't have as much equipment, I got to know the people there faster than at a large gym. An independent gym will be more attentive to their clientele, more friendly, and you might enjoy perks like free week-long guest passes for your friends, tips on exercising and a free session with a trainer (depending on the gym).

24 Hour Fitness is good because it's convenient with so many locations. Many of the members are young and single. They have a wide range of classes and (depending on the club) updated equipment.

Curves is great if you really value socializing with the workout. I often see women there chatting while they run in place and lift weights. If you're looking to maintain an easy workout program while you chat with others, Curves might be for you.

When you visit a gym, they'll give you a tour. Ask for a week pass to try out their gym. Don't settle for just a day. Insist on a week. This will give you plenty of time to get a realistic idea of whether the gym fits. Did you actually go? Is it a pain to get there at the time you'll most likely go? What about parking?

Classes or Sports Mini Guide

Since there are soooo many sports and classes out there, and I can't possibly cover them, the tips I can give are general:

- Call ahead to find out what you're going to need to bring and wear

- Bring a towel for sweat
- Bring a pen and paper or your cell phone to note down anything else you'll need to bring next time
- Bring a snack in case you get hungry and water, too
- Bring a friend if you're shy

It's time to get started!

Motivated Mover Activities to Try Today to Conquer the Details

---

ACTIVITY CHOICE: Incorporate these tip details into your exercise activities. Try a gym for a week if you haven't yet. You never know, you just might enjoy it.

TIP #9

Just Begin

There comes a time when the learning stops and the doing begins. This is that moment. Read this chapter. Thumb through the Appendices. And then commit here and now to our overall purpose mentioned in Tip #5:

Say to yourself, "**I will focus on fun when I exercise in some way, shape or form almost every day.**"

And then go take a walk...or skip...or somersault...just go move and make it fun!

In the end, it's simple. Just go for it.

Make that commitment to care enough about yourself, your health (mental and physical) and your well-being to exercise.

The rest—the goals, the drive—may come and go, but that purpose to have movement activities as a permanent part of your lifestyle will always remain.

So please, stop reading this book, close it up, pass it along to someone else who might need it, call up a friend, and move! That's all I ask. That's all your body ever asks.

Now is the time. Move.

Motivated Mover Activities to Try Today or Right Now to Just Begin

---

ACTIVITY CHOICE: Just do it. Close up the book and go for a walk at the least. Schedule your movement. Start today!

ACTIVITY CHOICE: Check out Appendix IV: Motivation Check-in. Make a copy of it and keep it close. When your motivation wavers, look at the check-in to discover where you still need to shore up your resolve. And if you still need a little more "oomph," check out the Bonus Tip.

BONUS TIP

Remember, When You Feel Ugly, Someone Else Makes Money

You've probably already heard this before, but at the risk of being boring, I wanted to remind you that when we feel ugly, it's often based on messages we have received from TV, magazines, movies and the Internet. When we feel ugly, someone makes a lot of money.

When we receive messages from advertising that we're "less than" or "ugly," and need to be fixed, we don't get angry. No. We feel ashamed. We feel bad until we give the companies (who told us we were ugly in the first place) money to help us fix our "ugly" problem.

Don't believe me? Okay. Let's look at the fashion industry. It's a billion dollar industry. How do they make their dough? Simple. By teaching us that we're "less than" unless we wear their clothes.

I can hear the fashion critics already: "Dahling it's so last season!"

Pharmaceutical companies have caught on, too. If someone doesn't have a lot of eyelashes, it's not a unique physical trait. It's *now a condition* called eyelash hypotrichosis. How do you fix it? Well easy, you buy their drugs!

How about the makeup industry? It earns billions by telling us we're almost perfect except for the following blemishes. Then they offer us the solution. Doesn't it sound so silly? And yet it works! Trust me, I know. Just ask my bank account!

The health and fitness industry is no better. The industry has done a great job of encouraging us all to regard any and all fat on our bodies as ugly. To rid ourselves of our "ugliness," we buy weight-loss programs. But the industry gives us the one-two punch because not only is fat "ugly," it has been turned into a "killer." To allow any excess fat to stay on our bodies is to assign ourselves an early death sentence. It drives us to buy health and fitness products like there's no tomorrow because we fear there IS no tomorrow.

Is Fat a Killer?

So is there no tomorrow for fat people? Do fat people really die earlier than the skinny ones?

To be honest with you, I am very confused on this topic. Here's why.

Most of us have heard about the "obesity epidemic." We've all heard that fat is bad. But what we don't hear is that the evidence often comes from studies funded by companies that profit from "fat is bad" results. Researchers who get funding from these companies sometimes find the results that help the companies gain profit.

I was surprised, too, to find data revealing the dangers of weight-loss, in particular when dieters yo-yo in their weight. Since it's reported that 75-80% of "weight losers" regain their weight back (and sometimes more) within three to five years of ending their diet, many of us are at risk. Here's why.

Yo-yoing in weight is called "weight cycling" by the medical community. Studies have shown that weight cycling three times with a loss of only 10 pounds can damage blood vessels and increase your cardiovascular risk. Weight cycling has also been associated with higher blood pressure and an increase of visceral (bad) fat. It is also strongly associated with increased risk for diabetes.

But weight cycling doesn't just damage us physically. It also damages us mentally. One study of teenagers found that dieting only serves to decrease self-esteem and coping mechanisms and encourage poor body image. If such negative consequences occur with our teens dieting, what makes us think it doesn't happen to us—at least on some level—too?

So why do we yo-yo?

Genetics plays a part. Studies show that how much we weigh is 45-81% genetics. In an article in the *New York Times* about current research in weight loss, it was suggested that "each individual has a genetically determined weight range spanning 30 pounds. Struggling against the brain's innate calorie counters, even strong-willed dieters make up for calories lost on one day with a few extra bites on the next. And they never realize it."

Evidence is mounting that fat may not be the killer we all think it is, either. Instead of approaching all fat as a killer, Dr. Glen Gaesser, doctor and author of *Big Fat Lies*, makes an argument for differentiating between bad fat (abdominal or visceral fat) and good fat (subcutaneous or near the skin fat). Visceral fat, due to its metabolic activity and makeup, is more likely to clog arteries, whereas subcutaneous fat is associated with counteracting visceral fat's damaging effects. Reducing one's intake of sugar and fat may help reduce the growth of visceral fat (bad fat).

Opposite from the mainstream argument that all fat is bad, several studies have associated fatter thighs with lower risks for cancers, high blood pressure, gallbladder and heart disease.

Given the difficulty of maintaining weight loss, the dangers of yo-yoing, and the findings that not all fat is bad, I wonder whether the "thin" messages we get from the media are actually more harmful than we think.

Studies estimate that as many as 40% of women in America are trying to lose weight at a given time (Methods for Voluntary Weight Loss and Control, NIH Technology Assessment

Conference Panel, *Annals of Internal Medicine* 1993). That's a lot of women...and a lot of money being thrown at diet programs, pills, foods and weight-loss methods that might bring more harm than good!

Hear It Once and Dismiss It. Hear It 1,000 Times and Believe It.

Maybe it's a little over the top to call these messages evil, but the impact to our psyches is very real, and the feelings of low self-worth can have a negative and long-lasting effect on the quality of our lives.

How effective are these messages?

Studies show that without body image education like this chapter, women are more susceptible to negative body images in the media. Researchers conducted a study with 1,000 college women and found that comparing idealized body images in the media with their own was connected with body dissatisfaction and lower self-esteem. After seeing idealized body images in the media, their body shame increased (Body dissatisfaction and body comparison with media images in males and females, *Body Image* 2007). These messages are not just affecting adult women. In one study, 83% of the teen girls interviewed wanted to lose weight even though 62% were in the Body Mass Index (BMI) "normal" range (Psychological and Physiologic Effects of Dieting in Adolescents. *South Med Journal* 2002).

Try this experiment if you'd like. Ask your girlfriends how they feel about their bodies. I bet that most will be unhappy with their bodies. I asked my friends, and true to form, almost all my vivacious and beautiful girlfriends wanted to lose weight or thought they were fat (including women who were far skinnier than I was). Most of them were on some sort of diet program.

It boggled my mind to realize how many of us are walking around, uncomfortable in our own skins. Don't we all deserve to feel comfortable in the bodies we have? Right now? Without having to fit into a certain shape or size?

Of course we deserve it!

So how do we begin accepting our bodies?

Body Acceptance Begins with Media Awareness

Wanting to improve our physical appearance is understandable. It's why we pay for good haircuts or get braces. We all want to feel and look attractive. It's only natural.

But you may not have to buy so much stuff to make that attractiveness come alive. Turns out, being your most attractive self is more of an inside fix than you might think.

Researchers have found that the more you receive body image education, the more you become satisfied with your body and the less you internalize society's beauty standards. Which means you'll be more confident. You'll hold your head up high. You'll shine from within.

Let's begin by limiting our exposure to media and being more aware of the messages they give us. I would recommend you start these activities today.

ACTIVITY CHOICES:

- Cultivate awareness of why you purchase products and why you might feel bad about your body or looks
- Circle spots on models in magazines you think are digitally enhanced or altered to remind yourself that even the models and actresses have a lot of help looking "beautiful." You can look up on the Internet "Photoshopped before and after photos" to get a good idea at how much images are altered.
- X-out any magazine image or message that makes you feel bad about how you look (make sure you own the magazine, though).
- Recognize the moment you begin to think you need to lose weight, count calories, etc. Was it the same moment Angelina came on the screen? Or a Dancing with the Stars professional dancer came on stage with half a dress on? Just take note.
- Choose non-advertisement entertainment (walk, run, skip, play games, read books, listen to music, etc.).
- Watch TV shows that make you feel good about your body (and mute or skip commercials).
- Read magazines that only make you feel good about your body. For example, try travel magazines that have nothing to do with body image or self-esteem, feminist magazines like BUST or even Oprah magazine can feature a larger variety of model sizes.
- Encourage positive body image talk with your friends instead of commiserating about fat thighs and stomachs.

This book is about accepting all body sizes, including those incredibly beautiful (by society's standards) models and actresses, so learn to extend compassion to the women you see in magazines and on TV. Women off-camera and without makeup look very different. Whenever you can, turn your eyes from the model in the magazine to the women you find walking down the street, in your exercise classes, your friends and family. Look for non-digitized beauty—what does it look like?

If you can, take this quote I found to heart: "Your body should carry you **to** your life's work. It shouldn't **be** your life's work."

Change Your Exercise Motivator and Get Comfy in Your Body

A lot of women begin exercising to lose weight—out of some combination of wanting to look good by society's standards and wanting to be healthier. I propose that if we're honest with ourselves, we'd say that our motivation heavily leans toward the "wanting to look good" side. That's perfectly fine. But it's difficult to maintain a lifetime of movement with that kind of motivator. Here's why.

A study showed that those who dieted and exercised to change their appearance were more likely to participate in drastic diets and were also more likely to fail than those who chose to change their lifestyle based on health. Feeling like we fail in the looks department (which just means we don't align with society's narrow beauty standards) is a very powerful negative motivator. Powerful negative motivators are like gusts of wind that billow a boat's sails but only for a few shaky moments. It's positive motivators that offer you the steady wind you need to move...and even change the course of your life forever.

If you truly believe you will be healthier when you're skinnier, check this out. In Linda Bacon's *Health at Every Size*, she found many studies showing our *activity-level counts much more than weight when aiming at living a long and vital life*. According to many doctors and eating disorder specialists, very few studies truly show that weight has any correlation to disease—until people get into the morbidly obese category.

I'd like to add that activity level also counts more than weight when aiming for happiness.

Many believe that body fat percentages and weight aren't true measures of health. Instead, blood pressure, blood cholesterol and blood sugar, along with fitness activity level, are a better indication of a healthy body.

If you still can't let go of weight, perhaps a better question than, "How do I lose 20 pounds?" should be the question Glen A. Gaesser suggests in *Big Fat Lies*: "At which weight do I feel most athletic and strong?"

I finally applied this quote to my life this year. I had been a vegetarian for a long time and switched to meat. Combined with a change in my schedule, I was eating more, exercising less and gaining weight. I was worried about it until I went hiking in Yosemite. And then I didn't worry about it again. I was ten pounds heavier. Having done the hike the year before, I had a clear memory of when I'd had to stop for breath. This time I felt the strongest ever. All the places where I rested before, I cruised by. I wouldn't exchange that feeling for anything—especially not some number on a scale.

My good friend recently changed the way she approached exercise, and I'm so proud of her. Before, she focused on losing weight, and the requirement of that goal was that she had to exercise. She could never sustain exercising for more than six weeks because the "wanting-to-look-good" motivator didn't sustain her. Exercise felt like punishment for being "overweight." But it didn't have to be a punishment for her. And it doesn't for you either. It can be used to strengthen your spirit and to make you feel good.

Now, she's focused on exercising as her goal. She's started looking into running and biking clubs. She switched her focus away from a weight-based program to a movement-based life, and she has succeeded in making exercise a more integral and enjoyable part of her life, instead of a chore.

The Body Positive, an organization promoting the Intuitive Health model, encourages a similar change in exercise motivation. They encourage exercising for fitness and release of mental stress. The shift in purpose supports a lifetime habit of physical fitness and health.

Accept Yourself and Just Move

If self-acceptance seems impossible, don't worry. We'll start with baby steps.

Baby Step 1: Become aware of the images you see that give you a negative feeling about your body. Every time you feel bad, note the feeling and what you're seeing around you. Acknowledge the feeling without judgment. If you feel like it, why not just say to yourself, "Nah, I don't believe I need to change a thing." Start today. If you like how it makes you feel, try a week of this. If you like how it makes you feel, try a month. And keep going!

Baby Step 2: A lot of women feel bad about their bodies. But where does it come from? Comments from friends and family? Media? Think about how you feel about your body, and your own history with your body image. According to The Body Positive, our poor body image can come from many places, "[It] may be anything from a single comment made by a peer that caused a woman to feel shame about her body, to the media's impossible beauty standards, to the story of an entire childhood that was centered around weight loss."

Baby Step 3: Instead of critically inspecting your appearance in every window you see, try a day where you must compliment something about your appearance.

Baby Step 4: If you're a consistent weigher, pack your scale in the closet for a week. No need to judge yourself with a number. If that's scary, try a day. See how you feel. If you feel liberated, perhaps you don't need the scale.

Baby Step 5: I mentioned this one earlier...but try it now if you like. Buy a women's magazine—whatever one you want—and a marker. Then write over every image you see in the magazine that has been digitally enhanced, makeup-enhanced, specially lighted, or has ads of extreme weight loss methods. I felt really free when I did this activity.

Baby Step 6: Create a positive ad about yourself. If you were a product, how would you convince someone to buy you? We can be really hard on ourselves. I felt really silly writing my ad, but when I was finished, I felt really good!

Baby Step 7: Go for a walk with only the intention of enjoying yourself. Feel your body and enjoy its ability to move. Go your own pace. Smell the roses, or rosemary nearby. Say hello to people you meet. Try for 10 to 20 minutes.

The whole point of this chapter is to jumpstart your body self-esteem. What our baby-steps can do is help us foster a confident, less susceptible body confidence that can take the idealized body messages we see with the ease of someone comfortable in her own skin.

If these baby steps have inspired you, check out the book *Transforming Body Image: Learning to Love the Body You Have* by Marcia Germaine Hutchinson, Ed.D. I highly recommend this book as a way to reconnect with your body.

On a final note, recently I was reading about media literacy and I loved this line: "Remember to be the person you want to be. You are beautiful. Ads should have people like you [in them]—you do not have to look like people in ads."

It's time for us to become who we have always wanted to be and let the influences of the world float by without us believing every word.

Motivated Mover Activities to Try Today or Right Now to Improve Your Body Self-Esteem

---

ACTIVITY CHOICE: Complete the baby steps suggested on the previous page.

ACTIVITY CHOICE: Simply sharpen your awareness of when you think poorly of your body and what triggers those thoughts.

Appendix I: A Sampling of Movement Activities You Could Try!

Backpacking

Baseball

Basketball

Bocce Ball

Body Building

Bowling

Boxing

Calisthenics (push-ups and crunches and pull-ups)

Canoeing

Catch or Pickle

Circuit training, sprinting, plyometrics

Climbing hills and hiking

Cricket

Cross country skiing

Cycling (outdoor or stationary)

Dancing

Fencing

Fishing

Flexibility (stretching, yoga)

Football

Frisbee golf

Gardening

Golfing

Gymnastics

Hackey sack

Handball

Hiking

Horseback Riding

Horseshoes

Kickball

Kickboxing

Lacrosse

Martial Arts

Nordic Trak (ski machine)

Pilates

Racquetball

Rock climbing

Rope jumping

Rowing

Rugby

Running

Sailing

Scuba Diving

Shuffle Board

Skating (inline or ice)

Skiing (water or snow)

Snow shoeing

Soccer

Speed, agility, and balance drills

Stair climbing

Step videos or other aerobic videos

Surfing

Swimming

Table tennis

Tai Chi

Tennis

Trampolining

Tubing and Bands

Ultimate Frisbee

Virtual sky diving

Volleyball

Walking

Water polo

Weight Training

Appendix II: Recommended Resources

Books

Health at Every Size: The Surprising Truth about Your Weight by Linda Bacon, PhD

"Fat isn't the problem. Dieting is the problem. A society that rejects anyone whose body shape or size doesn't match an impossible ideal is the problem. A medical establishment that equates 'thin' with 'healthy' is the problem. The solution? Health at Every Size." — excerpt from back cover

Big Fat Lies: The Truth about Your Weight and Your Health by Glenn A. Gaesser

"Here's proof that people can be overweight and still be fit and healthy." — excerpt from back cover

Transforming Body Image: Learning to Love the Body You Have by Marcia Germaine Hutchinson, Ed.D.

22 exercises brought to you by a licensed psychologist to walk you through the steps of becoming aware of your body and improving body image.

Women Afraid to Eat: Breaking Free in Today's Weight-Obsessed World by Frances M. Berg, MS

"'It's health at any size!' is this book's emphatic message to American women..." Berg, a licensed nutritionist, the founder/editor of

Healthy Weight Journal, and the author of several books, including *Afraid To Eat: Children and Teens in Weight Crisis*, argues that the media and society cause women to obsess over the numbers on the bathroom scale and subsequently abuse their bodies and minds." — excerpt from back cover

Great Shape: The First Fitness Guide for Large Women by Pat Lyons, Debby Burgard

- "Emphasizes the pleasure and enjoyment of an active, healthy life, rather than concentrating on losing weight
- "Describes walking, dancing, swimming, bicycling, aerobic activity, and includes valuable safety tips
- "Boosts self-esteem and restores self-confidence"
  — excerpt from back cover

Intuitive Eating: A Recovery Book for the Chronic Dieter by Evelyn Tribole and Elyse Resch

"Rediscover the pleasures of eating and rebuild your body image."
— excerpt from back cover

The Men's Health Gym Bible
by Myatt Murphy and Michael Mejia

"In The Men's Health Gym Bible, certified strength and conditioning coach Mike Mejia and magazine contributor Myatt Murphy instruct readers in the optimal use of a gym for strength training and cardiovascular fitness." — excerpt from back cover

AUTHOR'S NOTE: I know this is a guy's book but it's got a lot of good pictures and explanations and is a really great beginner's guide to resistance training and gym equipment.

Happiness is an Inside Job: Practicing for a Joyful Life by Sylvia Boorstein

"This book will convince you that your own happiness really is much more available to you than you may have thought."
—**Jon Kabat-Zinn, author of *Coming to Our Senses***

Web sites

Active at Any Size pamphlet:

www.win.niddk.nih.gov/publications/active.htm

AUTHOR'S NOTE: I don't like that they call this home page the Weight-control Information Network. I do think they have some valuable information on how to get started exercising regardless of body size or weight.

Body Positive

www.bodypositive.com

The Body Positive

www.thebodypositive.org

Appendix III: Meditation: We Only Have Now...and Now...
and Now. So Breathe.

Start by finding a quiet place. If you're already in a quiet place, take ten even breaths through your nose. In. Out. In. Out. Say a count in your head for every breath in if it helps. One...Two... Three... Focus on your breath and the sensation of the air entering and leaving your nostrils.

Did you do it?

How'd it go?

Did you feel even a smidgen more relaxed?

I hope so.

I tend to tense up my forehead and cheeks into a pretty good frown when I'm stressed. So, usually, the first muscles to relax are in my face. Then my shoulders relax. Sometimes I yawn. And my eyelids feel a tiny bit heavier.

So...did you think about stuff?

Now, take 10 more breaths and this time, when a thought appears, acknowledge it and then return your focus to your breathing. Try your best not to judge your thoughts.

You might wonder why we refocus on our breathing. First of all breathing is a consistent function of the body that we can feel, so it helps us stay present in our bodies. Secondly, our breathing is happening in the present moment. It is something we can concentrate on that is occurring now. Thirdly, it is a way to distance ourselves from our thoughts.

One of my favorite simple meditations is from Thich Nhat Hanh, a Vietnamese monk. As you breathe in and out, you think, "Breathing in, I feel calm. Breathing out, I smile." It can be simplified to simply thinking "calm" when you breathe in and "smile" when you breathe out. I have used this when I get into stressful situations like job interviews, doctor's visits, and traffic.

Appendix IV: Motivation Check-in

In spite of our best efforts, sometimes our motivation flags. We just can't seem to get ourselves to do any kind of exercise. Use this checklist to remind yourself of some of these key concepts and tips that can make all the difference. Put a check for every yes answer. Note where you didn't check yes and use that information to put your motivation back on track.

Is your activity fun?	☐
Are you paying attention to how great your body and mind feel after your exercise?	☐
Are you exercising at the best time of day?	☐
Are you getting bored with routine and need a refresher?	☐
Have you elected a mentor to help you?	☐
Have you done the walking meditation?	☐
Are you ignoring your excuses and getting to your exercise activity anyway?	☐
Have you tried the "lie to yourself" activity and promised a smaller workout?	☐
Have you scheduled your activity throughout the week?	☐
Do you have a goal that fits you?	☐
Are you fueling yourself properly?	☐
Are you talking nicely to yourself?	☐

Remember, the only time we fail is when we give up for good. Get back to exercising, find ways to make it fun, and keep going! You can do it!

Acknowledgements

I wanted to express my gratitude to those who made this book possible. Thank you to all the willing friends and family who found their way into this book as my examples of what real-life people do for fitness. Thanks to Ralph Liguori for his unwavering support of this project. Meredith Linden, thank you so much for your proofreading skills—if there is an error left, it is mine. To all my early draft readers: Tiff, Kell, Mom, Dad, Eric, Jeff, Trisha, and Jenn C. Thanks for striking that tough balance of kindness and honesty. Many, many thanks Jean, Shelly, Janet, and Linda for reading my book under a tight deadline and for believing in me. Jennifer, your expertise helped me move forward into the wild world of publishing. Thanks to Cindy Conners for life coaching me through my fears about publishing. And lastly, thanks to all my former clients who showed me how determination and a whole lot of joy can be transformative. Thank you.